Licensed Practical Nurse

GUIDE FOR EXCELLENCE

in Long-Term Care

Charlotte Eliopoulos
Specialist in Geriatric and
Long-Term Care Nursing

HEALTH EDUCATION NETWORK

CONTENTS

Foreword

The licensed practical nurse (LPN) in long term care increasingly faces more and more challenges. Indeed, the current nursing shortage has added to this dilemma. The LPN is faced with higher patient to nurse ratios, higher acuity of those patients, directing the activities of the certified nursing assistants (CNAs), and of course, the threat of malpractice. This book provides the LPN that for which they have not been trained. Having received their nursing education in some cases over a period of one year, one could hardly expect that they are prepared to meet the challenges with which they are faced in today's nursing facilities.

LPNs are usually described as not being able to assess patients, yet many do, and thus need education on how to proceed with this element of nursing. LPNs are not educated or trained on how to deal with and direct the activities of the CNAs, yet they are faced with this responsibility constantly, and thus need practical training in this area as well. Indeed, many are considered "supervisors" in the long term care facility. In their short period of nursing education, very little is presented in the area of legal liability. This book provides a clear and concise explanation of legal issues and provides examples of specific cases in so doing.

The delight of this book is that it provides a sense of respect and acknowledgement of the duties and responsibilities of the LPN, which is not usually apparent. Charlotte Eliopoulos presents the reader with a description of the professional opportunities awaiting the LPN who may consider working in a long term care facility, taking into consideration the challenge of providing care, in many cases independently, to nursing home residents who typically have multiple disorders. Add the fact that there is an opportunity to develop relationships with residents, this can be very attractive to LPNs. Throughout the book, the author approaches the education of the LPN with dignity, respect and a gentleness that one does not expect in an instructional text, especially a nursing instructional text. Furthermore, information which could be quite complex, is presented in an easy to understand manner, utilizing the use of examples, displays and illustrations.

Nursing home occupancy will experience much growth in years to come, as evidenced by the growing older population who will be in need of 24 hour care and supervision. According to the U.S. Bureau of Census, even though the rate of growth of the elderly will drop after 2030, there will still be a large population of elderly, a significant portion of which will need nursing home care. The need for quality education and development of the LPN will not go away, but will remain. The *Licensed Practical Nurse Guide for Excellence in Long-Term Care* satisfies those needs.

Joan C. Saunders
Founder and Executive Director
National Association of Nursing Administrators in Long-Term Care (NADONA/LTC)

Preface

This book is written for licensed practical/vocational nurses (LPNs) who are working in long-term care facilities. If you're one of these nurses you're among good company because more than one-fourth of all LPNS are employed in nursing home settings. You're also in a specialty that offers job security because there will be a continued demand for your services. According to the Bureau of Labor Statistics, the need for LPNs in long-term care settings is projected to grow faster than the demand in most other settings due to the growth of the elderly and disabled population that will need long-term care. Seems like you've made a wise career choice.

You're employment in a long-term care setting may not have been due so much to a planned career choice as to other factors. For instance, maybe there were no openings in the local hospital for LPNs but the nursing home was hiring, or perhaps there was a long-term care facility close to your home. Whatever the reasons that drew you to this setting, you're in a specialty that may allow you to use a wider range of nursing skills than many other settings where you could've been employed.

Perhaps you've noticed that we're using the term *specialty* to refer to long-term care nursing. Some people think that long-term care nursing is a watered-down version of acute care nursing–easier, less demanding, a piece of cake. In reality, nothing could be farther from the truth. Long-term care nursing requires unique knowledge and skills. The needs of chroni-

1

cally-ill individuals who reside in a facility are quite different from acute care patients who only have brief encounters with nurses. The relationships you share with residents and their families in the long-term care facility gives you a greater opportunity to be involved in holistic care—care that addresses physical, emotional, spiritual, and social needs—than nurses who work with people in short-term relationships. The type of staffing in long-term care facilities is hardly the same as other settings. Regulations and your role in meeting them differ from hospitals and home health. And often, you carry significantly more responsibilities and function more independently than LPNs in other settings.

It is foolish to think that in one year of education, LPNs can be expected to have obtained all the clinical and management skills that are required to be an expert long-term care nurse. To practice skillfully and competently in this specialty you need to add new knowledge and skills to your basic nursing education.

This book offers you the building blocks to prepare you for the specialty of nursing in a long-term care facility. It will cover the essentials of your role in this setting, such as how to:
- perform a comprehensive assessment
- develop and use effective care plans
- prevent and care for special clinical risks
- handle emergencies
- administer medications safely
- manage a team
- meet regulations and stay within the law
- grow in your role

There will be a lot of information presented in the pages that follow. We recommend you read a little at a time and give yourself a chance to fully absorb the content before moving on to a new section. Also, often it's helpful to discuss the content with an experienced long-term care nurse who can offer a perspective from having been there.

We commend you for taking this step to improving your knowledge and becoming the best long-term care nurse that you can be.

4

Licensed Practical Nurse

GUIDE FOR EXCELLENCE

in Long-Term Care

Chapter 1

INTRODUCTION TO
LONG-TERM CARE NURSING

This book was written for those special licensed practical nurses and licensed vocational nurses (we'll just use the term LPN for now on) who have chosen the path of working in a long-term care facility. We're going to assume you're one of them if you're reading this.

You really *are* special if you're working in a long-term care setting. You could be working in a more popular and glamorous field–and even one that pays better–yet you're working in a long-term care facility (LTCF). And it's great that you are because you fill an important role. RNs and physicians depend on you to carry out a variety of treatments and bedside care. Nursing assistants depend on you for direction and guidance. And, residents depend on you to help them get the care they need. Display 1-1 outlines some of the typical responsibilities of LPNs in LTCFs.

Pros and Cons of LTC Nursing

Why would you want to work in a nursing home?
Isn't that a depressing place to work?

It wouldn't be surprising if you've heard comments similar

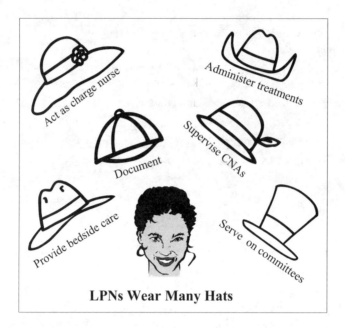

LPNs Wear Many Hats

to these when people learn where you work. Some people just can't understand your reasons for working in a LTCF. This attitude is understandable when you consider the image of nursing home care in society as a whole.

Most times, when the public hears about nursing homes on television or reads about them in the newspaper it is because there has been abuse, an injury, or some other bad event. Seldom do the many positive things that happen in LTCFs make the news. People begin to think that nursing homes are places where sick people are warehoused at the mercy of uncaring, cruel employees. The unfortunate actions by a few cast a negative light on all LTCFs.

The stigma that still plagues nursing homes, unfortunately, is a very real burden that you have to carry when you work in this setting. However, it is important to balance that against the positive aspects of working in long-term care.

Benefits of Working in Long-Term Care:

- *Independence:* Unlike hospitals and other settings where doctors and nurses are directing most of your actions, in the LTCF you get to make many of your own decisions and use your own judgment. The care is routine enough that you know what to expect and can feel secure in taking many actions on your own.

- *Relationship-centered care:* In some settings it seems that nurses spend most of their time hanging IV bottles, adjusting machines, checking monitors, and charting. The resident in the bed seems to get lost among all of the technical activities that must be done. But in the LTCF, you have the chance to interact with residents and to get to know every aspect of them. You become like family and make heart-to-heart connections that are just as important to care as the treatments that are done.

- *Holistic care:* Because the people you care for will spend a very long time in the facility in most cases, care must address the total person: body, mind, and spirit. You get to practice nursing as it was meant to be practiced.

- *Opportunity to use more skills:* Unlike other settings where LPNs are restricted in what they can do, in LTCFs you may carry some management responsibilities and perhaps do some teaching of the CNAs who you supervise. As a result, you get to use your talents and grow in your job.

Display 1-1
Responsibilities That LPNs Could Have
in Long-Term Care Facilities

Administrative

    Meets with members of the interdisciplinary team to assess, plan, coordinate, and evaluate residents' care.

    Documents nursing activities accurately and in a timely manner.

    Receives and records physicians' orders.

    Communicates staffing problems and needs to the unit nurse/supervisor.

    Develops work assignments for nursing assistants.

    Assure CNAs comply with job descriptions.

    Reports problems and complaints to the unit nurse/supervisor.

    Provides feedback to nurse managers regarding performance of nursing assistants.

    Receives and provides end of shift report.

    Assists in admission, transfer, and discharge of residents.

    Serves on and participates in committees as assigned.

    Assures CNAs comply with policies and procedures.

    Reports maintenance and housekeeping needs.

    Identifies and reports needs for supplies and equipment.

    Participates in the development, implementation, and evaluation of quality assurance activities.

    Adheres to professional codes of ethics.

Clinical

    Greets and helps to admit new residents.

    Makes rounds with physicians and other team members

    Assesses residents and assists in completion of the Minimum Data Set.

    Participates in developing, implementing, and revising residents' care plans.

    Coordinates residents' care activities.

    Identifies and reports changes in residents' status to physicians, responsible family members, and supervisory nurses

    Recommends, communicates, and implements changes in residents' care plans.

    Communicates care activities and changes to team members.

    Responds to emergency situations.

Communicates and coordinates care with residents and their families/significant others.
Administers treatments and other direct care.
Prepares and administers medications as prescribed.
Observes and evaluates residents' responses to medications.
Identifies and promptly reports adverse drug reactions.
Maintains narcotic records accurately.
Orders or arranges for ordering of pharmaceuticals.
Notifies physicians of automatic stop orders.
Notifies unit nurse/supervisor of discrepancies in drug inventories.
Collects specimens as ordered.
Implements restorative/rehabilitative nursing programs.
Respects residents' rights; protects residents from abuse and neglect.

Education

Communicates educational needs of staff to staff development coordinator and supervisors.
Participates in the orientation of new employees.
Provides instruction to staff as needed.
Provides education to residents and families.
Attends continuing education programs to maintain competency and improve knowledge and skills.

Public Relations

Promotes a positive image of long-term care nursing.
Meets with prospective/current residents and their families.
Promotes positive guest relations.
Assures problems and complaints involving nursing services are managed and resolved in a timely, appropriate manner.
Protects the privacy of residents and employees.
Represents the facility and nursing services in professional and community activities as assigned.
Maintains positive working relationships between nursing staff and other departments.

The responsibilities of the LPN can vary from facility to facility. Be sure to follow the job description for LPNs in your facility.

Understanding Residents

It's useful to understand the residents who you will meet in your daily work. Although you will find many different types of people in LTCFs, in general the nursing home population is

- *Old:* Over 90% of residents are over age 65; nearly half are over age 85
- *Female:* Among older residents women far outnumber men but among nonelderly residents the proportion of men equals that of women
- *White:* Minorities represent only 10% of the resident population
- *Alone:* Approximately two-thirds have no living relatives
- *Disabled:* Over 80% of residents need help with 3 or more activities of daily living. More than half are cognitively (mentally/intellectually) impaired

Being admitted to a LTCF is very different from being admitted to a hospital. Most people view hospitals as places where they go to improve and feel better. They know that the stay in the hospital will be brief and that the likelihood of returning home is strong. Their friends and families, knowing that the stay is limited and being familiar with hospitals, are likely to visit, send cards and flowers, and frequently ask about them.

Now, contrast the hospitalization experience with that of entering a LTCF. Most people enter a LTCF because they have conditions that are not going to improve and that will require care for the remainder of their lives (certainly this is not true for those entering for short-term rehabilitation, but these are in the minority). The views that their friends and families hold of LTCFs often are negative which cause them to not want to be there and their friends and families to dread having to visit

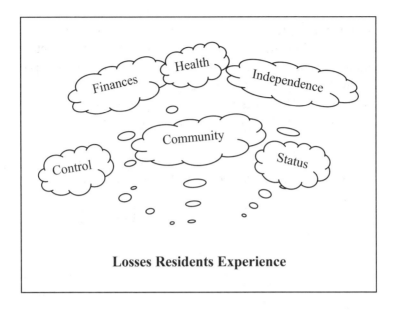

Losses Residents Experience

them there. Further, the reality is that as time goes on, visitors come less frequently and residents become less connected to their previous social world.

There are many losses that people face when they enter a LTCF. In addition to experiencing a loss of health, community residence, and contact with significant people in their lives, residents also face the loss of roles, status, independence, and finances. Coping with these losses as they adjust to their admission is a major task for residents, one that can trigger reactions such as:

Anger. Residents may be very critical of staff, food, and
the facility. This anger often is displaced onto staff.
Anger directed at family is common, also.

Depression. Residents may have a lack of interest in
food and activities; they may refuse to see their visitors.

Denial. Despite being told about the realities of their
conditions and the need for long-term placement, resi-

dents may make comments that make you wonder if they understand, such as "I'm only going to be here for a few weeks," and "I'm sure my daughter is trying to find a way to take me into her home."

Regression. Residents may not participate in their care as much as they are able and, instead, look to staff for assistance with activities that they could do on their own.

Reminiscing. Unable to cope with the realities of their present situation, residents may talk a lot about their past.

Fear. Residents may be suspicious of staff to the point that they cannot relax, or feel that they need to offer money to staff for proper treatment.

Your patience is needed by residents as they go through these reactions. Even if they are short with you or criticize you, remember that *it is the situation, not you, that they are unhappy with and that they are reacting to.* Allow residents to express their emotions. Be available to listen and lend support.

During their stay in the facility, residents will need the same careful attention to their care as residents in any setting. As will be discussed later in this book, there are some special care issues and risks that LTCF residents have that may be somewhat different from residents in other settings and there are some unique documentation requirements. In addition, and very importantly, there are *rights* that residents in LTCFs have, as required by law. If you haven't read the regulations pertaining to residents' rights, ask your supervisor for a copy of them. It is important that you be familiar with these rights because you have a responsibility for making sure that you and the staff that you supervise respect these rights. The next page lists some suggestions for promoting residents' rights.

Actions to Promote Residents Rights

- Allow maximum decision-making and participation in care.
- Assure residents understand diagnoses, plans, caregiving activities, changes, and services.
- Reinforce explanations given by physicians and administrators.
- Treat all residents with respect and dignity, without discrimination based on race, creed, color, religion, or source of payment.
- Inform residents when a change in room or roommate is anticipated and allow maximum resident participation in decisions pertaining to this change.
- Review assessment findings with residents to assure needs and priorities are viewed similarly between residents and staff.
- Request residents' input into care planning and delivery.
- Use nonrestraining means to control behavior (e.g., environmental modification, diversional activities, changes in approach).
- Offer explanations for the reason and importance of treatments and services without forcing residents to accept care that they want to refuse.
- Encourage and assist residents to use personal clothing.
- Assist residents in decorating their rooms with personal items.
- Afford privacy to residents and their visitors.
- Do not open or read residents' mail unless requested.
- Inform residents of the time and location of family and resident council meetings and assist them in participating in these meeting as necessary.
- Report residents' complaints to supervisory or administrative staff. If residents desire to report complaints to state regulatory agencies or other agencies, provide them with the necessary information regarding how to do so.

Families of Residents

Mr. and Mrs. Palo shared 40 years of a happy marriage when Mrs. Palo was diagnosed with Alzheimer's disease. The couple had never been apart and Mr. Palo vowed that he would care for his wife at home. However, keeping Mrs. Palo at home became more of a challenge than Mr. Palo bargained for. As Mrs. Palo's dementia progressed she would wander at all times of the day and night. Mr. Palo often had sleepless nights as he had to check on her and return her to bed during the night. She resisted bathing and could not be left alone. Things came to a head when Mr. Palo had to be hospitalized for a week and found that he had to juggle schedules with five different caregivers in order to provide 24-hour care for his wife. Physically and emotionally exhausted, Mr. Palo finally had to seek nursing home placement for his wife so that her needs could be met and his health wouldn't be threatened.

Mrs. Jefferson agreed to taker her mother, who had just had a stroke, into her home and provide care. Mrs. Jefferson's two brothers agreed to offer some financial help, but made it clear they could not assist in any caregiving. It didn't take long for problems to begin to surface. Mrs. Jefferson's mother, who had been a mild-mannered person, had developed an irritating, demanding personality after the stroke. Mrs. Jefferson was finding that she had less and less time for her husband and children. Mr. Jefferson resented the time and energy that his wife was spending on her mother and finally gave an ultimatum that his mother-in-law would have to leave or he would. Mrs. Jefferson approached her brothers to share in the care of their mother but they refused and suggested nursing home placement. Although this is not what she ever wanted to do, Mrs. Jefferson realized that she had no choice and located a nice facility not too far from her home. Hurt by what she saw as her children's unwillingness to care for her, Mrs. Jefferson's mother agreed to enter the facility, but told her children that she never wanted to see them again.

These are but a few examples of the roads some residents and their families travel as they make the decision for long-term care. Most residents are not admitted to a LTCF because they have uncaring families, but because their families cannot provide the care they need. Just think of your own life and imagine the adjustments you'd have to make if you suddenly had to provide hands-on care for a relative. Even with all your nursing skills, this would not be easy and, chances are, your entire life would be turned upside down.

Because families may have been down some rough roads before admission, they may not be at their best. When you meet them, families may be physically, emotionally, socially, and financially drained. They, too, need your patience and understanding.

Families also experience losses when their loved one enters a LTCF. Grandkids no longer can drop in and visit grandma for cookies and milk. A wife can no longer turn over in bed and feel the warmth of her husband. A daughter may have to be the one making decisions for her father instead of looking to her father for guidance. Families may grieve as a result of these losses and go through many of the emotions experienced with grieving, such as depression, denial, and anger.

It is not uncommon for families to feel guilty about having to have their relative in a LTCF. Perhaps they think that if they had only taken the person to the doctor's office sooner or if they had helped out more things wouldn't have gotten so bad. Or, maybe if they had only done more. This guilt can be increased by the resident's pleas to be taken home, angry outburst, and rejection. Even friends and neighbors can add to the guilt with comments like, "What a shame you couldn't find a way to keep your mother with you." Guilt can cause family members to be depressed and angry. Often, these feelings are displaced to staff through criticisms, unreasonable demands, and hostile outbursts.

Like residents, families need your patience and understanding. Some ways that you can help families are to:

- *Offer a listening ear and allow them to vent their feelings.* Reassure them that residents and families often have many feelings as they adjust to the LTCF and that things will get better with time.

- *Orient them to the facility.* Show them the location of restrooms, vending machines, telephones, and various offices. Describe the typical day for residents. Inform them of visiting hours. Give them the names of key staff that they can contact for questions or problems.

- *Suggest activities that they can do with the resident.* It is very difficult to be a visitor and spend visiting time just sitting next to the resident's bed. Recommend that they read, play cards, watch a movie, or work on a scrapbook with the resident during their visits.

- *Keep them informed.* Learning through the grapevine that their loved one fell or had an argument with another resident is unpleasant for families and can cause them to distrust staff. Avoid surprises by phoning them with information about unusual events or changes in status before they visit.

- *Welcome their input and feedback.* Let families know that you and they both want what's best for the resident and work

18

on the same team to achieve it. Invite them to attend or offer input into care planning conferences and to suggest ways to improve the resident's care.

Consider families your partners in care, not a bother. It helps to consider what you would want to be treated like if you were in their shoes!

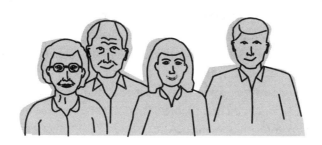

The "Team"

A wide range of talent is needed for a LTCF to operate. Each resident has needs for the proper diet, medications, treatments, medical attention, clean environment, and other services. Employees have needs to be trained, supervised, paid, and treated fairly. The physical structure has needs for maintenance and management. Regulators and insurance providers have needs for accurate documentation and data. To meet all these complex needs, the facility has many different departments:

Administration. There are considerable behind the scene activities that are required to keep a facility functioning, such as planning, budgeting, billing, purchasing, paying bills, communicating with outside agencies and investors, managing overall operations, and keeping the facility licensed. These activities are performed by the administrator/chief executive offi-

19

cer/president, fiscal officer, assistant administrators/vice presidents, accountants, bookkeepers, admissions coordinators, and other administrative staff. The governing body of the facility appoints an administrator to oversee day-to-day operations; in states where it is required, this person must be licensed. Typically, someone must be designated to assume the administrator's responsibilities when the administrator is not on the premises.

Nursing. As the need for nursing care is the primary reason for residents to enter a LTCF, this department is a vital one. Twenty-four hour nursing services must be provided to assure residents receive basic personal care, medications, treatments, and other direct assistance. A registered nurse must serve as a DON on a full-time basis. Nursing takes the lead role in coordinating resident care and services with other departments.

Medicine. All residents must have their own personal (attending) physician or a physician on staff of the facility to provide medical care. Physicians examine residents when they are admitted, develop a plan of care expressed in physicians' orders, visit residents as required, provide consultation and direction when there are changes in residents' conditions, and review the care on a regular basis. Physicians may delegate some of these responsibilities to a nurse practitioner. LTCFs must have a medical director who assures that all residents' medical needs are met, acts as a liaison with all attending physicians, and assures employees are free from infection.

Dietary. Because of the diversity of health conditions that the resident population can present, a variety of diets must be available. Meals must be planned to meet physicians' orders and be in accordance with the recommended daily allowances established by the Food and Nutrition Board of the National Research Council. Proper food storage, preparation, serving, and disposal are important responsibilities, particularly because problems resulting from the improper performance of these functions can be life-threatening.

Pharmacy. The number and range of medications administered to residents are considerable. Pharmaceutical services assure that drugs are properly ordered, stored, and administered. Although the facility is not required to have its own pharmacy on the premises, if it doesn't, it must contract for pharmacy services and arrange for a pharmacist to review each resident's medication schedule at least monthly. Only a licensed pharmacist can label and dispense drugs; only physicians, licensed nurses, and certified medication aides can administer drugs.

Activities. In addition to personal care and treatment of health conditions, residents need meaningful social, emotional, intellectual, and spiritual stimulation as they live in the facility. Music, art, dance, pet, and other therapies not only provide recreation, but can be therapeutic to physical, mental, and social health. The facility must provide an ongoing program of activities designed to meet the interests and needs of residents. This department is directed by a qualified therapeutic recreation specialist or an activities professional.

Social Services. Residents present a variety of social and emotional needs as they adjust to their illnesses and institutionalization. The facility must provide medically-related social services to assist in meeting these needs.

Housekeeping. A safe, sanitary environment is crucial in a facility in which ill, frail, and old people reside. This department maintains cleanliness and order in residents' rooms and other areas of the facility.

Laundry. Proper handling of linens is important in the prevention and control of infections. Laundry services may be provided as a department within the facility, as a component of the housekeeping department, or through a contract with an outside agency.

Maintenance. The physical plant and equipment are seldom given much thought—until they don't function. The maintenance department assures the proper operation of plumbing, electrical, heating, and mechanical systems, as well as facility compliance with the Life Safety Code of the national Fire Protection Association.

Medical Records. Documentation is a necessary evil in any health care institution. Properly maintained records are valuable in communicating important information about residents that promotes safe, consistent, and individualized care. The quality of these records can influence reimbursement, and, subsequently, the financial status of the facility. Also, in the event of litigation, the record serves as evidence of the events that transpired. In addition to organizing and storing residents' records, the medical records department may collect statistics that can guide the facility in its planning.

Human Resources/Personnel. In addition to caring for residents, the facility must care for its employees, too. The human resources or personnel department provides assistance in recruitment, reference checks, hiring, firing, disciplining, benefits management, and employee record maintenance. The expertise of this department can assure that the facility's labor practices are in compliance with the law and that employees are treated fairly.

Volunteers. These unpaid resources are valuable members of the facility. They often perform functions that staff lack the time to do and that contribute to a high quality of life for residents.

Other. Depending on the size of the facility, additional departments may exist, such as laboratory services, purchasing, central supply, and education.

None of these departments works in isolation. Each department's activities impact the others. Together they form a team that allows the facility to provide high quality services to residents and jobs to its employees. By understanding the function of all departments and respecting each of their contributions, you help to build a positive team spirit that helps the facility to function like a well-oiled machine.

Chapter 2

ASSESSMENT AND CARE PLANNING

Imagine that you are about to start a road trip across the country. You pack your bags, fill the gas tank, and jump in the car. Generally, you know the direction in which you need to go, but aren't quite sure which road to take as you have never traveled this route before. If you take Road A it may be going in the wrong direction, wasting your time and gas. Road B may be a dead end. Road C may put you on the Interstate, but then you'd miss some of the sights that you heard are great to see. *What do you do?*

It would be no surprise if you said that you'd never face this question because you'd have more sense than to start a road trip without a map and directions. It is the rare person who starts on a journey with no plan.

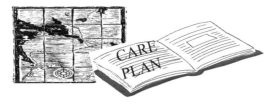

The journey of caregiving that you embark on with residents also needs clear directions to assure you reach your goal of quality, individualized care for residents. You need to know the destinations you need to reach and the actions you need to reach them. Also, and very importantly, you need to know about all aspects of the resident for whom care is going to be given and this is achieved through nursing assessment.

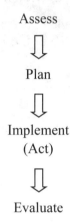

Assess

Plan

Implement
(Act)

Evaluate

Assessing Residents

You may have heard that assessment is the first step of the nursing process.

In addition to assessment being the basic foundation of nursing practice, it is required by law for LTCFs. The Omnibus Budget Reconciliation Act–the nursing home law that is commonly called *OBRA*– requires that residents be assessed at admission, whenever there is a significant change in status, and at least once within 12 months after their last assessment. As you know if you work in a LTCF, the assessment is documented on a standardized tool called the MDS (Minimum Data Set) that addresses the following areas:

cognitive status
functional status
sensory and physical impairments
nutritional status and requirements

special treatments and procedures
psychosocial status
dental status
medical conditions and their status
drug therapy
activities potential
rehabilitation potential
discharge potential

Usually, a RN performs and coordinates this assessment, however, LPNS often are asked to do parts of it. Because you may be asked to do some of the assessment for the MDS and you need to be able to assess changes in residents' status during your regular activities, it is important that you have good knowledge about this process. Following the areas on the MDS, let's review some of the knowledge you need to know to assess residents.

COGNITIVE PATTERNS

A **comatose state** is one in which the resident is in a state of deep unconsciousness, is unable to be aroused, and has diminished or absent reflexes. This condition can be a result of trauma, the ingestion of toxic substances, severe fluid and electrolyte imbalances, and disease such as hepatitis, cirrhosis, diabetes, and terminal cancer.

To assess:

- Observe mental and physical activity
- Attempt to arouse resident; call resident's name; give simple command
- Apply painful stimuli, such as pinching
- Determine bladder elimination; palpate for and note distended bladder
- Inspect eyes for corneal irritation (secondary to absence of corneal reflex)
- Review medical record
- Ask family members or significant others for information pertain-

ing to resident's level of consciousness, such as resident's norm, length of time in present state, their   observations of resident's reactions.

Cognitive status refers to the resident's memory, orientation, judgment, and problem-solving ability. Altered cognition is an abnormality and associated with a physical or mental health problem. A rapid onset of altered cognition typically is associated with a delirium, whereas the cognitive declines seen with dementias usually occur over a long period of time. Good baseline data concerning mental status are crucial in detecting changes in a timely fashion and assuring prompt treatment.

Memory loss is not a normal outcome of aging. Recall of events in the long past may be superior to recall of recent events for older adults, although this is believed to be more of a function of exercise of memory rather than a normal age-related decline. Alterations in short and long-term memory can be associated with physical or mental health problems.

The stress associated with admission to a health care facility can cause some residents to do poorly on their initial test of cognitive function. When alterations are noted, reassess the resident after he or she has had an opportunity to adapt to the new surroundings. Also, assure that hearing deficits aren't responsible for poor results on cognitive testing.

Normally residents should be oriented to their surroundings and be able to recall facts pertaining to person, place and time. When testing this area, assure that the resident has reason to know the information being asked. (For example, a resident may not have been outdoors for months and consequently may be unaware of the season.)

Normally the resident should display good judgment and be able to participate in daily activities with no problem. Sometimes, the stress associated with admission to a facility or   adjustment to a new situation can cause some difficulty in decision-making that often subsides as the resident adapts to the institutional setting.

Of the characteristics associated with dementia, impaired judgment, reduced coping ability, and hesitancy in making decisions or poor decision-making are present. This increases the risk of injuries and complications because the resident is less able to protect himself/herself, and places added responsibilities on staff to supervise and protect the resident.

To assess cognition:
- Tell the resident you are going to be stating three words for him or her to remember. State three simple unrelated words. As the resident to immediately recall the words.
- Continue with the interview. After five minutes ask the resident to state the three words given earlier.
- Ask the resident for information pertaining to the past, such as place born, schools attended, past presidents
- Ask "What is the season or time of the year?"
- Ask "What is this building that we are in?"
- Ask resident to identify his/her roommate, charge nurse, caregivers (Assure resident has been introduced to these persons)
- Take the resident to the hallway, dining room or other common area; ask the resident to return to his/her room or state its location
- Observe the resident's behaviors; note agitation, crying, inappropriate actions, reliance on others for basic decisions
- Determine judgment by asking the resident "What would you do if a fire began in the waste can in this room?" Resident should be able to give an appropriate response.
- Ask the resident to follow a simple three-stage command, such as "Pick up that piece of paper, fold it in half, and hand it to me."
- Note level of consciousness. Observe for restlessness, pacing, dullness, drowsiness.
- Assess speech: Is speech rational? Does the resident have difficulty finding the right work, or are inappropriate words substituted for intended ones? Can the resident state the name of familiar objects? Is speech slurred?
- Observe activity pattern.
- Describe pattern of cognitive function over a 24 hour period; use a flow chart to record observations.

- Compare findings pertaining to cognitive status to previous mental status evaluations if data available
- Ask resident and family about changes they have detected in resident's mental status over the past several months
- Evaluate vital signs; note abnormalities that could alter cognitive function, such as hypotension, hypothermia, hyperthermia, bradycardia
- Review resident's laboratory reports for indications of fluid and electrolyte imbalances, anemia, infection, and other problems that could alter cognitive state
- Review medications for drugs that could alter cognitive function, such an antipsychotics, antianxieties, anti-inflammatories, cardiac medications
- Review medical history for conditions that could alter cognitive function, such as cardiac problems, anemias, pneumonia, diabetes, fever, fecal impaction, hypoglycemia

Delirium is an acute state of confusion as a result of a disturbance to cerebral circulation. Problems such as infection, dehydration, hypoglycemia, adverse medication reactions, and cardiac, liver, respiratory, renal, or thyroid disorders can be the cause of delirious states. Cognitive function (memory, orientation, judgment) is impaired and there is an alteration in the level of consciousness ranging from mild drowsiness to hyper-activity. This confusional state has a rapid onset and usually is reversible upon correction of the underlying cause.

To assess:
- Note level of consciousness. Observe for restlessness, pacing, dullness, drowsiness.
- Assess speech: Is speech rational? Does the resident have difficulty fining the right word, or are inappropriate words substituted for intended ones? Can the resident state the name of familiar objects? Is speech slurred?
- Observe activity pattern.
- Describe pattern of cognitive function over a 24 hour period; use a

flow chart to record behavior and cognitive function hourly for at least the first day after altered cognitive function presents.
- Monitor vital signs, intake and output, general signs and symptoms.
- Review medications administered to resident over past week, laboratory data.
- Review history for recent loss, use of restraints, relocation; sensory deficits.

COMMUNICATION/HEARING PROBLEMS

Assessment of the resident's capacity to hear begins upon first contact with the resident. During the exchange of greetings the resident may display a tendency to cock the head to one side, rely on lip-reading and visual cues, ignore questions and comments, or ask to have things repeated. Further assessment can validate suspicions that a hearing deficit is present.

There are two general types of hearing problems that may be present. **Conductive hearing loss** stems from problems in the passage of sound through the canal, ossicles of the middle ear, or the tympanic membrane. **Sensorineural hearing loss** involves dysfunction of the inner ear receptors or the nerve itself. With aging, some degree of sensorineural loss often occurs; this is known as *presbycusis*. Since the higher frequency sounds are the first ones impaired in persons with presbycusis, special attention should be paid to avoid speaking to affected persons in a high-pitched voice, but instead, speaking loudly and deeply. Persons who have had exposures to loud noises have a higher risk of hearing problems; this emphasizes the importance of obtaining an occupational history from residents.

With age, the keratin in the cerumen is of a harder consistency and easily accumulates. Cerumen impactions can interfere with adequate hearing. The ears should be inspected for cerumen and if it is present, it should be removed.

To assess:
- Observe the resident for indications of lip-reading, cocking the head to one side, and requests to have things repeated
- Ask the resident if a hearing aid is or ever has been used

31

- Instruct the resident to use the hearing appliance during the assessment
- During the interview assess resident's ability to hear speech at various levels by:
    - asking a question in a whisper
    - placing your hand over your mouth while asking a questions
    - getting behind the resident or turning your back and asking a question
- Hold a watch to each of the resident's ears and determine the ability to hear the ticking
- If a hearing appliance is used by the resident ask:
    - How long have you used the hearing appliance?
    - Where did you obtain the hearing appliance/who prescribed it?
    - How do you care for the appliance?
    - What problems do you have using the appliance?
    - Are you able to hear speech and environmental sounds clearly with the appliance?
- Examine the hearing appliance for condition, cleanliness, function
- Inspect the resident's ears for cerumen accumulation and foreign matter
- If hearing deficit is noted, review record to determine date of last audiometric examination; consult with the unit nurse or physician to arrange audiometric examination if one has not been conducted in past year
- Ask the resident how the hearing deficit has impacted activities of daily living, social activities, role
- Ask the resident to describe effective means of communicating with him/her

Effective communication allows residents to understand and enjoy their soundings, share emotions, participate in activities, and protect themselves from threats to their health and well-being.

Communication problems can stem from neurological conditions, altered mental status, adverse drug reactions, and disease of the ears, nose, and throat. Astute assessment can assist in identifying the underlying cause of the communication problem. During the assessment, attention should be paid to the phase of communication that is impaired; for instance, is the problem *receptive* (difficulty hearing, seeing, interpreting, understanding), *expressive* (difficulty selecting appropriate word, forming sentences, forming words, writing, and using nonverbal means of expression), or *global* (total inability to understand, formulate words or express self)? The ability to understand and express oneself in written words is an important area to assess, also. Throughout the assessment of communication ability, consideration must be given to the resident's education level and competency in using the English language.

To assess:

- Observe the resident's reaction to conversation and questions: Does resident have little or no change in facial expression? Are directions and questions understood? Are appropriate responses and behaviors displayed?
- Ask the resident to perform a simple task, (e.g., "Please pick up that glass of water") to determine if a receptive problem exists.
- Write a simple question on a piece of paper, give it to the resident, and ask him/her to answer it (e.g., "What is your first name?"); if a problem exists, determine if it is a result of the resident not understanding the written question or the inability to form or articulate the answer. *Dyslexia* is the term used to describe problems in reading material. .
- Ask the resident and family members or significant others if there has been any change in the resident's communication pattern over the past few months. If problems have been noted, ask about other symptoms that may be present or factors that may have contributed to the problem (e.g., new medication, recent infection, mood change).
- When comprehension problems are apparent, determine to what extent they are present, e.g., understands most of the time, understands if instructions are broken into simple steps, does not understand at all. Ask family members and significant others for

33

their assessment of the resident's understanding.

- Inquire about mechanisms resident has used to facilitate communication, such as communication boards, pad and pencil, synthesizers.

VISION PATTERNS

Vision impairments are common findings among nursing home residents. Much of the reason for this has to do with the fact that most residents are advanced age, and the eye experiences many changes with aging. One of the basic and most common changes is the reduction in accommodation power of the eyes that causes difficulty in seeing small objects closely, known as *presbyopia*. Corrective lenses are required to correct presbyopia, and since this process is progressive, eyeglasses often need to be strengthened every several years.

There is increased opacity of the lens; some degree of *cataract formation* exists in virtually all older persons. This can cause vision to appear hazy and increase sensitivity to glare.

Peripheral vision (to the side) is reduced with age. This problem is more profound in residents with glaucoma. Residents who have experienced a CVA may have a reduction in the same half of the visual field of both eyes, known as *homonymous hemianopsia*. Persons with *macular degeneration* lose of central vision.

Other age-related changes can be noted. A yellowing of the lens can occur, making it more difficult for older eyes to discriminate among various shades in the color groups of blues, greens and violets. Corneal sensitivity is lessened, thereby reducing the older resident's ability to detect irritation and infection in a timely manner. The resident may complain of seeing spots floating across the visual field, a nonpathological, although annoying, outcome of aging called *vitreous floaters*. (The number and size of these spots should be discussed with the resident because spots that are large, of great number, or of recent onset could be associated with retinal disease.) Weakening of the structures around the orbit can cause the eyelids to turn in (*entropian*) or turn out (*ectropian*). The eyes lose some of their luster. A grayish ring at the outer border of the cornea may be seen, called corneal arcus or arcus senilis; this does not affect vision. More time is required for older eyes to adapt from dark to light, and vice versa.

Seeing flashes of light, or halos or rings around light is an abnormality associated with a variety of conditions, such as glaucoma and digitalis toxicity. Seeing something that is not present (hallucination) or misinterpreting something that is present for something that is not there (illusion) is associated with emotional disturbances; when these problems exist it is important to determine if the problem is psychiatric or a result of sensory deficits, adverse drug reactions, or other factors.

To assess:

- Inspect the eyes for redness, tearing, dryness, turning in (*entropian*) or out (*ectropian*) of the eyelid, yellow sclera, infection, lesions, drooping of the eyelid over the area of the pupil (*ptosis*).
- If the resident has eyeglasses or contact lenses, assure they are worn during the assessment.
- Ask about the date of the last eye examination and where eyeglasses were obtained; review medical record for information concerning date of last eye exam. Refer resident for if it has been ≥ 1 year since opthalmological exam
- Ask about the use of eye medications. If resident has been using drops for glaucoma management, assure they are ordered and continued without interruption (abrupt discontinuation could cause an increase in intraocular pressure).
- Ask about sensitivity to glare, problems with certain types of lighting, difficulty with vision in dark areas or at night.
- Ask resident about symptoms, changes, and problems related to eyes and vision. For example: Has your ability to read/see things at a distance/see things clearly changed? Are your glasses strong enough? Do you have any blind areas in your vision? Do your eyes ache or pain? Do you ever see flashes of light or halos or rainbows around lights? Have you been bumping into things lately?
- Use a newspaper to obtain a gross assessment of the resident's visual acuity. Ask resident to read the headlines and progressively move to the smallest print; describe the specific size of newsprint that resident is able to see (e.g., "Can see only headline-size print

matter"; "Able to read small newsprint using eyeglasses.")

- If resident is unable to read headlines on newspaper, determine if resident can see and follow your finger; if resident cannot do this, determine gross visual capacity (e.g., "Can make out shapes"; Able to differentiate dark and light, but cannot see objects"; "No vision".)
- Review with resident measures used to compensate for visual deficits, e.g., use a large print books and magnifying glasses, wearing sunglasses when in bright areas, placing objects on right side to compensate for poor left-sided vision.

MOOD AND BEHAVIOR PATTERNS

Mood and behavioral problems are not uncommon in the long-term care setting. Multiple losses, role changes, adjustment to institutional living, and poor health status are among the factors causing mood alteration to be present in many residents. Depression, agitation, and chronic complaining may be noted in residents who suffer mood alterations. Alzheimer's disease and other dementias also can be responsible for mood and behavior problems.

Mood and behavior changes can be detected through obvious signs, such as crying, cursing, hitting, and verbal expressions. However, subtle signs can be present and must be observed for; these include: disinterest in appearance, refusal to participate in activities, increased dependency, reduced food intake, and resistance to care.

Many mood and behavioral problems are reversible, thus, a comprehensive review of contributing/causative factors is essential. Areas to review include administration of new drug, fluid and electrolyte imbalances, sensory deficits, hypo/hypertension, relocation, and changes in routines/staff.

To assess:

- Review the resident's medical history and assessment of cognitive patterns for problems that could affect mood and behavior.
- Observe the resident (during routine activities) for: crying, angry outbursts, handwringing, pacing, repetitive behaviors, wandering, arguing, cursing, hitting, scratching, shoving, inappropriate sexual comments or behaviors, smearing or throwing food or feces,

screaming, self-abusive acts
- If problem behaviors or mood alterations are noted:
  - identify pattern, intensity, duration, frequency, onset
  - explore precipitating or related factors, (e.g., wandering increased when unit is noisy, becomes agitated when lights are turned off, argues with staff who attempt to have resident perform ADLs independently)
  - interview resident and family/significant others to determine if this is new problem or a lifelong pattern (e.g., resident may have come from family or neighborhood in which violence was an acceptable means to deal with problems, resident may chronically use threat of suicide to get attention)
  - determine impact on resident's safety and well-being
  - determine impact of resident on others
  - ask resident for self-assessment of how mood or behavior affects his/her life
- Note food intake; if warranted, record percentage of each meal consumed
- Observe for hoarding of medication
- Observe for refusal to take medications, have treatments done, or participate in activities. Determine if there is any legitimate reason for the refusal
- Observe and ask staff about resident's activity pattern and initiative in activities
- Question resident about mood, feelings of hopelessness, considerations of suicide. If resident admits to having thought about suicide, ask if he/she has ever considered how it could be accomplished. (Note: Resident who have planned or attempted suicide should receive evaluation.)
- Review resident's history for need for restraints (physical or chemical) to control behaviors and circumstances in which they were used.
- Review for environmental factors that could affect mood and behavior (e.g., noise, poor lighting, lack of privacy, cold temperatures,

unstable staffing change in routine, relocation).
- Review medications for those that can alter mood, such as: psychotropics, antihypertensives, digitalis, steroids, sedatives, stimulants, immunosuppressives, cytoxic agents
- Review medical history and laboratory tests for conditions that can alter mood and behavior, such as dementia, depression, cancer, hypercalcemia, hypoglycemia, CVA, sensory impairments, or thyroid, cardiac or Parkinson's disease

PSYCHOSOCIAL WELL-BEING

The resident's current psychosocial status must be put in perspective of the resident's lifelong pattern. Persons who had troubled relationships through life may be more likely to have conflict with other residents and staff. Likewise, persons who avoided group activities and had few friendships, may be the "loners" in the facility.

Techniques such as life review and reminiscence therapy can assist residents in reflecting on their past and putting their current status into perspective. By encouraging discussions of residents' past roles and activities, staff can promote psychosocial well-being in residents.

To assess:
- Review assessment data for cognition, communication patterns, and physical functioning and structural problems for factors that could interfere with psychosocial well-being (e.g., dementia, impaired hearing, restricted mobility).
- Interview resident and family/significant others to learn about recent changes or losses in resident's life, resident's past patterns of friendships and social activities.
- Ask the resident to tell you a brief history of his/her life and describe what he/she believes to be major accomplishments.
- Ask the resident how he/she feels about being in the facility, the staff, other residents.
- Ask resident to describe the role that religious/spiritual beliefs play in his/her life.
- Observe resident for:
  - ease of interacting with other residents and staff

38

- nature of verbal interactions (e.g., friendly greetings, angry out-bursts)
- frequency of visitors, nature of visitations
- participation in activities (willingly participates, needs coaxing)
- mood, body language
- Compare resident's current physical and mental ability to partici-pate in activities to that of the past; identify factors that impacted resident's past level of psychosocial function; determine degree to which current roles, status lifestyle conflict with that existing pre-admission.
- Explore losses that could be causing resident to grieve and how grief is being managed (e.g., having to give up pet, death of friend, inability to be active in community, no longer able to be caregiver for spouse, needing to sell family home).

PHYSICAL FUNCTION
AND STRUCTURAL PROBLEMS

Regardless of the medical diagnoses that residents possess, it is their level of function that most affects the quality of daily life and directs nursing activities. An assessment of physical function is es-sential to planning care appropriately, maximizing resident's inde-pendence and minimizing risks to health and well-being.

Physical function can be determined in several ways. Medical diagnosis can yield insight into functional capacity. During their physical examination of residents, nurses learn about structural and functional problems. Evaluation of residents' performance of the activities of daily living (ADL) provides relevant information on resi-dents' level of independence in meeting the basic self-care needs of eating, bathing, dressing, toileting, continence, and mobility. An as-sessment of instrumental activities of daily living (IADL) promotes an understanding of how well people can perform activities that enable them to be independent in the community (e.g., housekeeping, cook-ing, shopping, handling finances, using a telephone, taking medica-tions, and traveling in public); since IADL evaluation provides in-sights most useful in determining how people function in the commu-nity, it tends not to be done in the long-term care setting unless it is

39

relevant to discharge planning activities.

The section of the MDS that addresses physical function is concerned with residents' performance of ADL (bed mobility, transfer, locomotion, dressing, eating, toilet use, personal hygiene, and bathing). A two-step evaluation is done for each of the ADL. First, the *self-performance* of the resident in meeting the specific task is assessed. This is followed by a determination of the ADL *support provided* by staff for each of the ADL. The period of time upon which the ADL assessment is based is the last 7 days, over all shifts. To gain an accurate assessment and assure the input of all shifts, the use of a flow chart, upon which every shift rates ADL function and assistance required, can prove beneficial.

Paralysis, weakness, shortness of breath, missing limbs, pain, and other physical condition can affect ADL function. Likewise, ADL limitations can be associated with mental impairments, such as dementias and depressions. Consideration also must be given to other factors that limit ADL performance, such as adjustment to a new environment, lack of knowledge of the facility's routine, and inability to locate materials needed to perform self-care tasks. Barriers to independent function should be eliminated.

CONTINENCE

Many older residents display changes in their elimination patterns as a result of the aging process. Urinary frequency is perhaps one of the most obvious of these changes and is a result of reduced bladder capacity. Reduced muscle tone can lead to some residual urine after voiding—a factor contributing to UTI. Constipation tends to be highly prevalent, and is associated with decreased peristalsis, insufficient fiber and fluid intake, and limited activity; many of the medications that residents take are highly constipating, also.

Incontinence is an abnormality, but one that is common in nursing home residents. (Approximately one-half of all residents are estimated to suffer some degree of incontinence.) The causes of incontinence are many, and include infections, poor muscle tone, bladder outlet obstructions, neurological disease, medications, altered mental status, and dependence on others for toileting. Incontinence can be categorized as follows:

- *Stress:* Caused by weak supporting pelvic muscles. When pressure is placed on the pelvic floor (e.g., from laughing, sneezing, coughing) there is an involuntary loss of urine.
- *Urgency:* Due to urinary tract infection, enlargement of the prostate, diverticulities, or tumors of the pelvic or bladder. Irritation or spasms of the bladder wall cause a sudden elimination of urine.
- *Overflow:* Associated with bladder neck obstructions and medications. Bladder muscles fail to contract or periurethral muscles do not relax, leading to an excessive accumulation of urine in the bladder.
- *Neurogenic:* Arising from cerebral cortex lesions, multiple sclerosis and other disturbances along the neural pathway. There is an inability to sense the urge to void or control urine flow.
- *Functional:* Caused by dementia, disabilities that prevent independent toileting, sedation, inaccessible bathroom, or any other factor that interferes with the ability to reach a commode.

A thorough evaluation is warranted when incontinence is present, particularly since many causes of incontinence are correctable, thereby causing the incontinence to be reversible.

It should be remembered that incontinence may be a hidden problem in some residents. Some persons may be reluctant or embarrassed to discuss this problem, and observation during the assessment can aid in exposing incontinence. Sensitivity in discussing incontinence is important, also. For example, the resident's incontinence should not be discussed in the presence of visitors or other residents, and incontinence briefs or pads should not be referred to as "diapers".

To assess:

- Review the medical history for problems that could contribute to incontinence, such as delirium, dementia, depression, CVA, diabetes mellitus, congestive heart failure, and UTI.
- Review assessment data related to resident's cognitive patterns and

physical functioning and structural problems for problems that could contribute to incontinence or affect Review medications resident is taking for those that can affect continence, including: diuretics (particularly furosemide, bumetanide, metolozone), antianxiety drugs, sedatives, anti-psychotics, antidepressants, narcotics, anti-parkinsonism agents, antispasmotics, antihistamines, calcium channel blockers, alpha blockers and alpha stimulants

- Note odors, stained clothing, and other indicators of incontinence
- Ask the resident about presence of incontinence by using questions such as:
  - Do you have any problem with bladder or bowel control?
  - Do you ever dribble urine?
  - Do you leak urine when you cough or sneeze?
  - Do you ever wet during the night?
  - Do you have problems reaching the toilet in time?
  - Can you sense the urge to void?
  - Do you ever need to wear a pad or special undergarment to contain urine?
- Inspect, percuss, and palpate the abdomen for bladder fullness, pain, or abnormalities.
- If an incontinence problem exists, ask the resident:
  - How long has incontinence been present? When did it begin?
  - Did the incontinence accompany another problem or event, such as start of a new medication, relocation, constipation?
  - How often does it occur? Every time? Only at night?
  - What amount is released? A large amount? A few drops?
  - Does it occur in relationship to other factors or events, e.g., after meals, when excited?
  - Do you feel the urge to void or is urine just released with no notice?
  - Do you have enough time to reach the toilet after sensing the need to void?
  - Can you toilet independently? What type of help do you need?
  - How does incontinence affect your activities, your lifestyle?

- Assess the resident's reaction to incontinence. (e.g., does he/she accept it under the belief that it is normal with advanced age, is he/she socially isolated due to embarrassment over the condition?)
- Consult with the unit nurse about having the resident who is incontinent checked for fecal impaction
- A post-void resident (PVR) may be ordered to assist in the resident's evaluation: After the resident has voided normally, measure the urine. Within 15 minutes of the voiding, catheterize (with a non-indwelling catheter) and measure the residual urine. Maintain sterile technique throughout the procedure. If the resident is incontinent, observe when voiding occurs and catheterize within 15 minutes.
- If the resident is incontinent, assure a recent clean catch or sterile urine specimen has been sent to the lab for evaluation.
- Discuss positive findings for incontinence with the unit nurse or physician to determine the need for further diagnostic evaluation. Obtain the physician's opinion as to the potential for continence.
- Establish the resident's normal pattern of bladder and bowel elimination by asking the resident about the normal pattern or maintaining an elimination record (flowsheet) for several days.
- Identify factors that could interfere with the resident's continence, such as inability to ambulate independently, not remembering location of bathroom.
- Ask resident or family/caregivers for information regarding incontinence control products or approaches that have been effectively used.
- Ask resident or family/caregivers if any change in continence has been noted in the past 90 days; describe the change.

HEALTH CONDITIONS
To assess:
- Review resident's record for any new problem in past week, including:
  - altered bowel elimination
  - dizziness/vertigo/syncope

- edema
- changes in vital signs, weight
- pain
- shortness of breath, coking, productive coughing
- vomiting
- confusion
- hallucinations/delusions
- tarry or bloody stools, hemoptysis, hematuria
- Review resident's record and incident/accident reports for falls, fractures or other accidents in last 6 months
- Ask resident and direct care staff about new health problems and accidents
- Observe and question resident about bowel elimination in past week; if constipation or diarrhea-like stool is noted, assess for fecal impaction
- Perform range of motion on all joints of resident; note new limitations, pain.
- Observe resident changing positions and ambulating. Note new limitations, pain, fatigue, dizziness, instability.
- Inspect and palpate for edema. Ask resident if puffiness has been noted, shoes and rings feel tighter.
- Observe resident's respirations; if difficulties are noted, listen to lungs.
- If problems are discovered, explore for factors that could have caused/contributed to new health condition, and determine impact of problems on physical and mental function.
- If resident has fallen in past 6 month, review care plan for measures to prevent falls and evaluate effectiveness of those measures.

ORAL / NUTRITIONAL STATUS

There is a direct relationship between nutrition and general health status. Good physical and mental health promotes a good dietary intake; in turn, ingesting the correct nutrients can keep individuals active and healthy.

Maintaining a good nutritional state can be particularly problematic for nursing home residents. By virtue of the fact that they need long-term care, residents have health problems and altered function that can interfere with their ability to meet nutritional needs. Medications can affect appetite and the energy level required to eat well. Weakness, pain limited use of one's body can threaten nutritional intake, as can depression, dementia and other alterations in mental or emotional status. The institutional food can be very different from the ethnic foods enjoyed by some residents and cause a reduction in food consumption. Also, most of these residents are of advanced age, and age-related changes can significantly alter nutritional state; for instance:

- food may taste different due to a decrease in the number of functioning taste buds (the most significant losses involve the buds for sweet and salty flavors)
- although tooth loss is *not* a normal consequence of aging, most of today's elderly wear dentures, thereby affecting the chewing and taste of foods
- food moves down the esophagus more slowly and remains in the stomach for a longer period of time, giving a sense of fullness after meals and increasing the risk for aspiration
- indigestion problems increase due to poorer food breakdown, intolerances to fatty and fried foods, delayed gastric emptying
- slower peristalsis, low fiber intake, and inactivity are among the factors that cause constipation to be a common occurrence
- the sense of thirst is decreased, which can interfere with residents drinking adequate fluids to protect themselves from dehydration
- older bodies have less total body fluid, thereby reducing the safety margin for dehydration

Although caloric needs are reduced in late life, the calories that are ingested must be of a good quality. Vitamin requirements remain the same in late life as in younger years. Protein intake should range between 0.5 to 1.0 g/kg daily. Various studies suggest calcium intake requirements from 850 to 1020 mg per day. Fluid intake should be at least 1500 ml daily, unless contraindicated.

When assessing residents, it is important to review all factors that impact nutritional status or that *could potentially* cause nutritional problems. Close, ongoing monitoring of nutritional status and observation for clinical signs of malnutrition are essential. **Clinical signs of malnutrition** include:

- weight loss
- dull, dry hair; hair loss
- dark circles under eyes
- dry, flaky, or scaling skin
- poor skin turgor (since skin turgor can be poor in many older residents due to reduced skin elasticity this can be an unreliable sign; however, skin turgor is best maintained over the sternum and forehead areas, thus testing over these areas may yield more usable data)
- swollen face
- pale, dry eyes
- red, swollen lips; fissures at corner of mouth
- tongue that is swollen, raw, bright red, smooth, or "hairy" looking; fissures, sores or white patches on tongue
- bleeding gums
- dry, rough, flaking, broken, or swollen skin
- hypo- or hyperpigmented skin; petechiae
- brittle, ridged, or spoon-shaped nails
- muscle atrophy
- weakness; confusion

ORAL / DENTAL STATUS

Tooth loss is *not* a normal consequence of growing old, however, a history of poor oral hygiene, environmental influences, poor nutrition, and changes in gingival tissue are factors that contribute to a high degree of tooth loss among older persons. Dentures commonly are present. The faster rate of bone loss in the lower jaw of edentulous individuals and changes in tissue structures can lead to dentures fitting

46

less well and needing to be adjusted every several years. Teeth that are present often are found to be brittle due to increased calcification; pieces of teeth can break off while residents eat and lead to aspiration, as a result. Poor dental care, a high carbohydrate diet, and insufficient intake of calcium can influence the development of caries.

All residents require careful attention to oral hygiene. Teeth should be brushed and flossed daily; special equipment is available to assist disabled persons to independently perform these functions. Residents with dentures should cleanse the dentures daily and brush their gums with a soft brush to remove debris and stimulate circulation to the gums. Nursing staff should regularly inspect the oral cavities of residents to assure cleanliness and intact mucous membrane, and to detect problems in a timely manner. Also, evaluation of every resident's ongoing ability to independently provide good oral hygiene is important.

Examine the oral cavity (wearing gloves throughout the examination):

- Inspect the oral cavity; use a flashlight and tongue depressor to assist.
- Note the presence of debris and general cleanliness.
- Observe the condition of the mucous membrane; note color, moisture and integrity of the membrane. If irritation or sores are present ask the resident how long the problem has been there and try to determine the causative/contributing factor (e.g., friction from poor fitting denture. [*White patches resembling dried beads of mild could indicate moniliasis infection; brown pigmentation in light-skinned persons can occur with Addison's disease; bright red spots encased by hyperkeratotic epithelium, on the hard palate, may be nicotine stomatitis; dryness can reflect dehydration]*
- Detect unusual breath odors; describe as precisely as possible. [*Sweet, fruity breath occurs with ketoacidosis; urine odor to breath can be associated with uremic acidosis; clover-like breath may accompany liver failure; and an extremely foul odor to breath can reflect halitosis or a lung abscess]*
- If dentures are present, examine for proper fit. Ask the resident to

remove the dentures and note condition.
- Inspect the gums. Note discoloration, inflammation, bleeding. [*Swollen gums can be associated with dilantin therapy or leukemia; red, bleeding, swollen gums can occur with periodontal disease; a bluish, black line along the gumline can develop from lead, mercury, or arsenic poisoning*]
- Refer for dental consultation if problems are noted or resident has not had dental examination in more than one year.

SKIN CONDITION

The skin requires good circulation to stay healthy and intact; unfortunately, this requirement is a challenge for many residents. Many residents have limited mobility, leading to extended pressure on the tissue, and consequently tissue hypoxia. Age-related changes to the skin made the skin more fragile and sensitive, Since many resident's possess factors that make them high risk for skin problems, it is important to regularly inspect the status of the skin, including areas hidden by shoes or clothing. Consideration should be given to the aggressive prevention of skin problems.

To assess:
- Observe the general status of the skin. Ask the resident to remove clothing and examine all surfaces of the body. Note color, cleanliness, moisture, temperature and abnormalities. (Dry, flaky skin, know as *ash,* can be a normal finding in black-skinned individuals and may be assisted by moisturizers.)
- Ask about itching, burning or other symptoms. If symptoms are present, question as to how long symptoms have been present, pattern (e.g., all the time, worsens at night). Review history to determine factors that could be associated with symptoms (e.g., exposure to pet, use of new soap, stress).
- Using the back of your hands, touch the cheeks and extremities of the resident to obtain a gross assessment of skin temperature. Note inequalities between sides. [*With stasis ulcer, the affected extremity will feel cool, although it may look red and inflamed, poor circulation can cause coolness of the skin surface.*]

48

- Test skin turgor by gently pinching various areas of the skin. (Since many older persons have decreased turgor due to age-related changes, poor turgor is a common finding. However, the skin over the sternum and forehead areas tends to lose less turgor than other areas, thus these are good areas to test.)
- If lesions are present, describe them in as much detail as possible in relation to: color, shape, size, and presence of drainage.
- If pressure ulcer is present, describe exact location, size (measure diameter and depth), stage, and drainage. A photograph of the ulcer may be useful as a means to accurately record the status of the ulcer and evaluate progress.
- Review record for history of resolved/cured pressure ulcers, descriptions of skin care measures, special treatments, etc.
- Review resident's diagnoses and assessment data for factors that make resident high risk for skin problems (e.g., infection, diabetes mellitus, CVA, dementia, poor sensations)

ACTIVITY PURSUIT PATTERNS

Participation in activities has multiple physical, psychological and social benefits to residents. However, maintaining an active state can be difficult for many residents due to their health problems and advanced age. Special encouragement and assistance may be necessary to promote residents' participation in activities.

When assessing activity patterns in residents, it is important to put current preferences and patterns into perspective in regard to those of the past. Some individuals live a life full of activities: they play sports, travel, entertain friends, have hobbies, and participate in community functions. Other persons are content with more passive activities: they may prefer staying at home alone, reading a book or watching television, and doing as little as possible. Understanding past activity patterns is invaluable to planning meaningful activities and identifying problems. For instance, refusal to participate in group functions and preference to be along in one's own room can reflect a problem for the person who was gregarious and engaged in many activities while in the community; on the other hand, such behavior in an individual who was a "loner" who enjoyed passive interests would not necessarily be viewed as abnormal.

It is important to remember that solitude is as important as social interaction. Every human being needs some time alone. This can be difficult to achieve in the institutional setting, however, quiet time and respect of privacy should be promoted to the fullest degree possible.

Individual patterns for rest and sleep can exit as well. In general, it can be expected that older residents will need a shorter block of night-time sleep (5-7 hours should be sufficient) and short naps during the day. Residents who sleep excessively may be suffering from health problems, such as depression or cardiopulmonary disease, or may be reacting to medications (e.g., sedatives, psychotropics, antihyperten-sives, analgesics).

To assess:

- Observe resident's rest and sleep pattern. The use of a flow chart to record rest/sleep patterns over a 24 –hour period can be benefi-cial. Consult with staff on all shifts for information about resi-dent's pattern.
- Observe for and ask resident about quality of sleep. Specifically ask about: breathing difficulties while sleeping pain, muscle spasms, nightmares, need for toileting, interruptions
- Identify factors that could influence sleep/rest pattern (e.g., medi-cations, unit noise, lighting, lack of meaningful activities).
- Ask resident to describe activities that promote rest and sleep (e.g., warm drink at bedtime, backrub, music, reading).
- Review medical record and interview resident to identify factors that could interfere with activities, such as:
  - physical or structural impairments
  - embarrassment about use of equipment, appliances
  - changes in role/status/self-concept
- Explore external factors that could interfere with an active state (e.g., unit layout, insufficient planned activities, lack of peers with comparable levels of function, overprotection by staff or family, demanding treatment schedule, inadequate staff to provide assis-tance).

MEDICATION USE

Medication use in nursing home residents is a serious and complex area of practice. Among the reasons for this are:

- the high number of drugs prescribed: an average of six drugs are administered to each resident daily, with some residents consuming considerably more
- the type of drugs prescribed: the most commonly prescribed drugs are cardiovascular agents, antihypertensives, analgesics, antiarthritic drugs, psychotropics, laxatives and antacids. Many of these drugs carry the risk for severe side effects and adverse reactions
- age-related differences in the way older residents absorb, metabolize, and excrete drugs

Due to the high risk for medication-related complications, careful assessment is essential.

To assess:

- Review all medications that the resident is taking. Note:
  - reason for drug is prescribed
  - attempts to manage problem without drugs
  - dosage and its appropriateness (i.e., Is it aged-adjusted?)
  - frequency of administration
  - if PRN, specific indications for use
  - number of psychotropic drugs prescribed
  - evaluation of effectiveness of drugs
- Ask the resident if he/she notices any positive or negative effects from drugs (e.g., improved mood, dry mouth, excessive drowsiness, better coping).
- Review resident's history for signs and symptoms that could indicate adverse drug reactions, such as:
  - blood pressure declines: psychotropics can cause postural hypotension
  - high fever: psychotropics can interfere with temperature regulation
  - altered cognition, mood, or behavior
  - declines in physical function or self-care capacity
  - appetite changes

51

- profound sedation
- dizziness, syncope, falls
- **anticholinergic symptoms:** dry mouth, confusion, constipation, disorientation, urinary retention, fever, blurred vision, hallucinations, insomnia, agitation, restlessness, picking behavior, short-term memory loss
- **extrapyramidal symptoms:**
    - Parkinsonism: tremors, postural unsteadiness, rigidity of muscles in limbs, neck and trunk, pill-rolling motion with fingers, shuffling gait)
    - akinesia: decrease in spontaneous movement)
    - dystonia: holding neck or trunk in rigid, unnatural position, e.g., turned to one side or hyperextended
    - akathisia: inability to be still
    - tardive dyskinesia: thrusting movements of tongue; lip smacking, puckering, or chewing movements; abnormal limb movements
- Assess resident for postural hypotension: Measure blood pressure while resident is lying down. Have resident stand for 5 minutes and measure blood pressure again. (If resident is unable to stand, measure while resident is in sitting position.) Blood pressure drops of more than 20 mm Hg are abnormal. Report abnormal findings.

Monitor resident's behavior and mood to evaluate effectiveness of psychotropic drugs. (Remember that several weeks of therapy is necessary before results are noted.) If drug does not appear to be effective or is causing adverse reactions discuss with physician.

SPECIAL TREATMENTS AND PROCEDURES

A special procedure included in this section is the use of restraints. Studies have shown that as many as 40% of nursing home residents are physically restrained for reasons ranging from controlling wandering to preventing falls to managing aggressiveness. Many serious consequences can result from restraint use, including strangulation, contractures, incontinence, pressure ulcer development, and poor self-concept. The unnecessary and excessive use of restraints lead to a heightened emphasis on the cautious use of these devices in the current federal regulations which states that *"the resident has the right to be free from physical or chemical restraints imposed for the purposes of discipline or convenience and not required to treat the resident's medical condition"* (from OBRA).

Anything that restricts the resident's movements is considered a restraint and includes: protective vests, geri chairs, trays on wheelchairs, safety bars, bedrails, safety belts

Restraints should be used only after other nonstraining alternatives have proven unsuccessful. There should be documentation describing the other approaches used. Review the resident's record for special care and therapies that have been performed.

Be sure to report changes in a resident's status as soon as you notice them.

Care Planning

A good assessment will reveal the resident's problems and needs that require attention. The care plan describes what staff need to do to address these issues. Care plans are required by law so it is important that they be done. However, the most important reason for developing a care plan is to provide that road map for care that we discussed earlier. Care plans must be working tools and to do so it is important that they be:

- *accessible.* A well-written care plan, neatly filed in a resident's record or book at the nursing station may impress surveyors, but it could have little meaning to the staff that care for residents. Certainly, you need to assure that an acceptable document exists to satisfy documentation requirements, but it is important that staff have access to the information. This can be done by making copies of care plans that can be kept in a book that is easily available to staff and by creating pocket-sized cards that provide the highlights of nursing-related aspects of the care plan that can be given to staff at the beginning of the shift and returned with when staff give their end-of-shift reports.

- *understandable.* Terminology needs to be clear enough to be understood by every caregiver. Don't assume that because staff should know certain medical terms, that they actually do.
- *specific.* A caregiver who is unfamiliar with a resident may not understand what "increase fluid intake" or "toilet frequently" means for a given resident. Clearer guidance is offered by stating "assure the resident consumes at least 600 ml on day and evening shifts" and "take resident to the bathroom every 2 hours during 8AM and 9PM.
- *reinforced.* If no one bothers to ask if the care on the plan was given or if the plan needs to be altered, staff easily can get the impression that this tool has little meaning.

Discuss goals and actions with CNAs to assess what they know about the plan, and ask if the goals and actions are meaningful.

Chapter 3

SPECIAL CLINICAL ISSUES

The characteristics of LTCF residents—old, frail, with multiple health conditions—cause them to be at high risk for complications. Nursing staff need to be proactive in preventing these complications. Let's take a look at some of the common clinical risks and actions that can be taken to reduce them.

Falls

Some studies have shown that a majority of nursing home residents experience a fall each year. These falls can cause injuries that lead to disability and death. Even if serious physical injury doesn't occur, emotional damage can result from a fall in that residents who fall may feel depressed and helpless, and be afraid to engage in activities.

There are several reasons that lead to the high rate of falls in residents, including:

- *Age:* Most residents are old and have experienced age-related changes that put them at risk for falls. These changes include reduced vision, poor night vision, less foot and toe lift during stepping, slower responses, urinary frequency that causes increased trips to the bathroom, and changes in the center of gravity which causes balance to be easily lost.

- *Improper use of mobility aids:* Canes, walkers, and wheel-chairs, although helpful, can be a safety risk if improperly used.
- *Medications:* Common drugs used in the facility (e.g., antipsychotics, diuretics, sedatives, antihypertensives) can cause dizziness, drowsiness, incontinence, and other problems that increase fall risk
- *Symptoms:* Confusion, dizziness, weakness, fatigue, unsteady gait, and edema often accompany some of the diseases that are common among residents. These symptoms can cause residents to fall more easily.
- *Unsafe clothing:* Poor-fitting shoes and long robes and pants legs can cause residents to trip and fall.
- *Environmental hazards:* Residents can slip on wet surfaces and waxed floors, and trip over linens and other objects left on the floor. Poor lighting also can contribute to falls.
- *Caregiver actions:* If caregivers do not respond to call-lights in a reasonable time frame, residents may try to get out of bed on their own. Poor supervision of residents who are unsteady on their feet or who are confused, failure to lock wheelchairs during transfers, and improper use of restraints can lead to falls.

It is important to identify residents who are at high risk for falls and actively prevent them from falling. Display 3-1 offers some tips on reducing the risk for falls.

Display 3-1
Reducing the Risk for Falls

- Identify residents who are at high risk for falls. These could include those with:
    - cognitive impairment, confusion
    - depression
    - hypotension
    - paralysis
    - muscle weakness or tremors
    - unsteady gait
    - immobility
    - seizure disorders
    - impaired vision
    - incontinence
    - a history of falling
    - and those who:
        - take many medications
        - use cane, walkers, or wheelchairs
        - are of advanced age
- Offer assistance to residents with toileting, transfer, and ambulation as needed
- Remind residents to use handrails and change positions slowly
- Clean spills promptly
- Avoid the use of restraints
- When a fall occurs:
    - keep the resident immobile until examined
    - if there is any possibility of a fracture, make sure that the resident obtains an x-ray
    - even if the resident is believed to be free from injury, monitor carefully after the fall because some injuries are not apparent immediately
    - complete an Incident and Accident form according to your facility's procedure

Infections

There are many factors that add to the high risk for infection in LTCF residents, such as:

- an age-related decline in the immune system's function
- the many chronic conditions that residents have
- age-related changes to body systems (e.g., enlarged prostate, increased fragility of skin, weaker bladder muscles)
- living in an institutional setting with exposure to a variety of people.

Immunization of residents and staff aids in preventing some infections. Upon admission, all residents should be asked about immunizations.

Pneumococcal vaccination is recommended for all residents unless contraindicated; reasons to not give this vaccine include pregnancy, lactation, and in some cases, immunosuppressive therapy and Hodgkin's disease. Although a single lifetime vaccination typically is recommended, revaccination may be considered after five years in people at high risk.

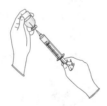

Influenza immunization is offered yearly, usually in the fall, although newly admitted residents can be immunized at any time during the flu season. Influenza immunization is repeated annually. Contraindications include egg allergy and pregnancy (first trimester).

Tetanus toxoid should be offered every ten years and can be repeated in five years if a dirty wound is sustained.

Display 3-2
Standard Precautions

- Handwashing when in contact with resident or resident's blood, body fluids, secretions, excretions, and contaminated equipment and articles; after removing gloves; before contact with other residents

- Use of gloves when in contact with resident's mucous membranes, nonintact skin, blood, body fluids, secretions, excretions, and contaminated items.

- Use of mask, eye protection, face shield when there is any risk of splash or sprays from blood, body fluids, secretions, and excretions.

- Wearing gown during procedures when there is risk of splashing or spraying blood, body fluids, secretions, and excretions.

- Protection of skin and mucous membrane exposure, contamination of clothing, and transfer of microorganisms to other residents when handling linens and equipment used by a resident.

- Proper cleaning and processing of reusable equipment.

- Routine cleaning and disinfection of resident's furniture and environmental surfaces.

- Disposal of used needles and other sharp objects in puncture-resistant, labeled sharps container.

- Avoidance of mouth-to-mouth resuscitation; use of mouthpiece, resuscitation bag, or other ventilation device.

- Use of private room if resident cannot maintain proper hygienic practices or if there is risk of resident contaminating environment.

A physician's order and the resident's consent
are required for immunizations.

Antibiotics have helped to control infections that would have been fatal in the past. However, the increasing and sometimes overuse of antibiotics have created a new set of problems in that some strains of bacteria have become resistant to antibiotics. It is important that antibiotics not be overprescribed.

Standard Precautions are used in the care of all residents as a means to prevent the spread of infection. Display 3-2 describes these precautions.

Pressure Ulcers

It is the rare resident who isn't old, malnourished, immobile, or with a health condition that affects skin status, so it's wise to consider all residents at risk for pressure ulcer development and to assure that some plan is in place to prevent this complication.

Remember that residents who are out of bed in a chair
also can be at high risk for developing a pressure ulcer
and that a q2h turning schedule may not be frequent
enough for some residents.

When residents do have pressure ulcers, assure aggressive treatment is implemented. If these ulcers were acquired from a hospital or other source, be sure this fact is clearly noted in the residents' records. Assure treatment orders are followed and that the documentation indicates the regular objective measurements, staging (Display 3-3), and other related factors.

Display 3-3
Staging of Pressure Ulcers

Stage 1: persistent area of skin redness that does not disappear when pressure is relieved; no break in skin

Stage 2: partial-thickness loss of skin layers that presents as an abrasion, blister, or shallow crater; no necrotic areas

Stage 3: full thickness loss of skin that exposes the subcutaneous tissues; looks like a deep crater without or without undermining adjacent tissue

Stage 4: full thickness loss of skin and subcutaneous tissue; muscle and/or bone exposed

Dehydration

Like pressure ulcers, the characteristics of LTCF residents make them at high risk for developing this complication. Unless medically contraindicated, residents need to consume at least 1200 ml (preferably 1500 ml) daily.

Clinical signs of dehydration can be tricky to detect because they easily can be confused with other conditions or aging changes. For example, the dry, inelastic skin of many older residents can prevent poor skin turgor (elasticity) from being a sign that can be used to detect dehydration. The confusion, weakness, and lethargy that occur with dehydration can be mistaken to be caused by other existing conditions. You need to be on the lookout for subtle changes—e.g., a worsening of confusion, weakness that prevents participation in activities that presented no problem in the past—and to report them promptly. Other signs of dehydration include:

- elevated temperature and pulse
- decreased BP

- reduced urinary output
- increased concentration of urine
- BUN $\geq$60mg/dL

Urinary Incontinence

As you probably know if you're working in a LTCF, incontinence is a common finding among residents. About half of all residents have urinary incontinence. The causes of incontinence are many, and include infections, poor muscle tone, bladder outlet obstructions, neurological disease, medications, altered mental status, and dependence on others for toileting.

It is important that the resident be thoroughly evaluated when incontinence is present, particularly since many causes of incontinence are correctable and bladder control can be restored.

Incontinence may be a hidden problem in some residents. Some persons may be reluctant or embarrassed to discuss this problem, so your observations during care help in identifying incontinence. Sensitivity in discussing incontinence is important, also. For example, the resident's incontinence should not be discussed in the presence of visitors or other residents, and incontinence briefs or pads should not be referred to as "diapers". Some measures to help incontinent residents include:

- Assuring the reason for the incontinence has been
  properly identified
- Collecting information about voiding pattern that can
  help in the assessment, such as voiding times, signs
  and symptoms accompanying voiding (e.g., pain, burning, lack of awareness that voiding has occurred),
  amount voided, characteristics of urine, and resident's
  reaction (e.g., distressed, unaware)
- Monitoring intake and output

- Assuring toileting facilities or bedpans/urinals are easily accessible
- Providing assistance with toileting as needed
- Implementing a bladder retraining program if it has been determined that the resident can regain bladder control:

Bladder Retraining Program

- Review record and consult with unit nurse, physician or nurse practitioner to learn of resident's potential to regain bladder control
- Explain procedure to resident
- Assure all caregivers are aware of the plan and are following it consistently
- Encourage good fluid intake
- Maintain a record of the resident's voiding pattern (time, amount, awareness of need to void, ability to reach commode in time, ability to control elimination, related factors)
- Determine the average time the resident can hold urine before becoming incontinent
- Remind or assist resident to toilet approximately 30 minutes before anticipated time to void
- Encourage voiding by running water, pouring small amount of water over vulva or penis, massaging over bladder
- Offer praise for appropriate toileting
- If resident is incontinent between scheduled voiding times, evaluate cause
- Document outcomes

- Implementing a prompted voiding program if the resident is unable to regain bladder control:

Prompted Voiding

- Determine the resident's voiding pattern and anticipated time of voiding

- Regularly ask or check resident for wetness/dryness
- Instruct resident to void or toilet resident before anticipated time of voiding
- Offer praise for successful toileting
- Provide adult briefs and other urine containment products as needed
- Assure skin is kept clean and dry (remind caregivers to cleanse resident's skin thoroughly after each incontinent episode as urine salts that dry on skin can be irritating)
- Clean urine spills promptly to prevent falls, keep path to bathroom/commode obstacle-free
- Assure resident has good fluid intake (fluid intake can be reduced in the evening but fluids shouldn't be eliminated entirely in the evening)
- Respect resident's privacy; do not discuss incontinence or check for wetness in presence of others
- Avoid indwelling catheter use if at all possible; if they must be used, follow procedure for care to prevent infections

Fecal Impaction

Granted, they are not exciting topics for conversation, however, fecal impactions are among the major events that demand your attention. The high risk for constipation among many residents causes fecal impactions to be a problem that easily can develop. Once they develop, fecal impactions easily can be missed because the liquid material that oozes around the impactions can be mistaken for diarrhea.

Prevention certainly is the best management of fecal impactions. Instructing CNAs to keep an accurate record of bowel elimination and reviewing these records can significantly aid in detecting and correcting constipation promptly.

Once a fecal impaction has developed, it must be softened,

broken, and removed. Sometimes oil retention enemas are used to dislodge the impaction. Manual breaking and removal of the feces with a lubricated gloved finger and injecting 50 mol of hydrogen peroxide through a rectal tube can assist with removal, also. Do not attempt to remove these impactions on your own. Your department should have a policy describing nurses' responsibilities in removing fecal impactions.

Changes in Mental Status

There is a high number of residents with Alzheimer's disease and other dementias in most LTCFs. In fact, there are so many residents with cognitive impairments that one could think that mental decline was a feature of growing old. However, dementia is not a normal state at any age. A decline in cognitive abilities usually means something is wrong.

Display 3-4   Possible Causes of Delirium

Fluid and electrolyte imbalances	CNS disturbances
	Emotional stress
Medications	Pain
Congestive heart failure	Malnutrition
Hyperglycemia and hypoglycemia	Dehydration
	Anemias
Hyperthermia and hypothermia	Infection
	Hypotension
Hypercalcemia and hypocalcemia	Trauma
	Malignancy
Hypothyroidism	Alcoholism
Decreased cardiac function	Hypoxia
Decreased respiratory function	Toxic substances
Decreased renal function	

There are two major types of changes in mental status that you may find among residents: delirium and dementia. *Delirium* is a rapid change in mental status caused by conditions that can impair circulation to the brain. Display 3-4 lists some of those conditions.

Signs that can be displayed with deliriums include:

- disturbed intellectual function
- disorientation of time and place but usually not of identity
- altered attention span
- worsened memory
- fluctuating mood
- meaningless chatter
- poor judgment
- altered level of consciousness, from hyperactivity to mild drowsiness to a semicomatose status
- disturbances in sleep-wake cycles
- suspiciousness
- personality changes
- physical signs, such as shortness of breath, fatigue, and slower movements.

Prompt action is needed when residents develop deliriums. By correcting the underlying cause, mental function can be restored in most situations. Also, treatment of the underlying conditions can avoid a worsening of the underlying conditions which can lead to complications.

Dementias are the permanent changes in mental status caused by diseases that injure the brain. Alzheimer's disease is the most common of these. Dementias are slow in developing and the lost mental function cannot be regained. Many of the signs associated with delirium are present in the resident with a dementia. Usually, there is not a change in level of consciousness in the resident with dementia.

There are times when residents with dementia develop deliriums. This can happen if they get an infection or other condition that disrupts their body function. Because they are confused to start with, it can be hard to detect the onset of delirium in a resident with a dementia. Caregivers who are familiar with the resident may be in the best position to see the little changes of worsened mental function and should be encouraged to report these changes.

Most of the care required by residents with dementia falls within the scope of nursing practice. One of the major considerations is the safety of these residents. Their poor judgment and misperceptions can lead to serious behavioral problems and mishaps. A safe, structured environment is essential. Caregivers and the location of items in the environment should be consistent. Items to trigger memory are useful to include, such as photographs of the resident or a consistently used symbol (eg, flower, triangle) on the bedroom door or personal items. Noise, activity and lighting levels can overstimulate the resident and further decrease function; therefore, they need to be controlled. This is particularly useful in preventing and managing sundowner syndrome (see Display 3-5). Cleaning solutions, pesticides, medications, and nonedible items that could be ingested accidentally must be stored in locked cabinets. Coverings should be applied to unused sockets, electrical outlets, fans, motors, and other items into which fingers may be poked. Matches and lighters should not be accessible; if the resident smokes, it must be under close supervision. Windows and doors can be protected with Plexiglas, and nonremovable screens can be installed to avoid falls from windows.

Wandering is common among residents

with dementia; rather than restrain or restrict them, it is better to provide a safe area in which they can wander. Protective gates can be installed to prevent residents from wandering away; alarms and bells on doors can signal when they are attempting to exit. With the great risk of residents wandering away and not being able to give their names or residence when found, it is crucial to have ID bracelets on them at all times and a recent photo available.

Various therapies and activities can be offered to the resident with dementia, depending on the resident's level of function. Occupational therapy and expressive therapies can benefit those with early dementia. Various degrees of reality orientation, ranging from daily groups to reminding the resident who he or she is during every interaction, can be used. Even the most regressed resident can maintain contact and derive stimulation through activities such as listening to music and touching various objects. Being touched is also a pleasurable and stimulating experience.

The physical care needs of residents with dementia can easily be overlooked. These individuals may not complain that they are hungry, so no one notices that they have consumed less than one quarter of the food served; they cannot remember to drink water, so they become dehydrated; they fight their bath so strongly that they are left unbathed; and pressure ulcers on their buttocks go unnoticed. These residents need close observation and careful attention to their physical needs. Thought must be given to the fact that they may be unable to communicate their needs and discomforts; a subtle change in behavior or function, a facial grimace, or repeated touching of a body part may give clues that a problem exists. This reinforces the importance of having the same caregivers assigned to these residents because they will be familiar with a resident's unique behaviors and more quickly recognize a deviation from that

Display 3-5
Sundowner Syndrome

Residents with dementias may have a worsening of behavioral problems when evening comes. This evening/night confusion is called sundowner syndrome because it occurs "after the sun goes down." Some of the factors that increase the risk of this condition include unfamiliar environment (e.g., recent admission to a facility), disturbed sleep patterns (e.g., from sleep apnea), use of restraints, excess sensory stimulation, sensory deprivation, or change in circadian rhythms. You can help residents with sundowner syndrome by:

- Placing familiar objects in the resident's room.

- Providing physical activity in the afternoon to help the energy to be spent.

- Adjusting lighting to prevent the room from becoming dark in the evening.

- Keeping a nightlight on throughout the night.

- Having frequent contact with the resident to offer reassurance and orientation.

- Using touch to provide human contact and to calm the resident.

- Assuring the environmental temperature is within a comfortable range.

- Controlling noise and traffic flow in the evening.

- Assuring the resident's basic needs are met (e.g., adequate fluids, toileting, dry clothing) individual's norm.

As residents regress, their dignity, personal worth, freedom, and individuality may be jeopardized. Loved ones may view the demented family member as a stranger living inside the body that once housed the person they knew. Staff sees another dependent or total-care resident before them with no sense of that person's unique life history. Viewed less and less as a normal human being or as the same person that has been known, the person with dementia may be treated in a dehumanizing manner. Special attention must be paid to maintaining and promoting individuality, maximum independence, dignity, and connection with other people.

Behavioral Problems

It's not uncommon to have residents who have behaviors that disrupt the entire unit. These behavioral problems are not only disruptive, but can threaten the safety and well-being of the resident and other people on the unit.

A variety of factors can cause or worsen behavioral problems. These can include:

Dementia

Delirium

Pain

Fatigue

Adverse drug reactions

Misperceptions of the environment due to
 sensory impairments or mental illness

Stress

Changes in routines, caregivers, health status

Increased dependence

Boredom, inactivity

When a resident shows behavioral problems, it is important to try to find out the reason. To help in the assessment of behavioral problems, observe and describe the following as precisely as you can:

Actions, behaviors that are disruptive

Time of onset

Where it occurred

Environmental conditions (dark area, noisy, cold)

People present

Events that occurred before onset

Length of time behavior lasted

Measures that helped or worsened the behavior

Outcome

A review of these factors can help the interdisciplinary team in identifying possible causes for the problem and ways to correct it. For example, if a resident became loud and threatening when his roommate had several visitors in the room, a plan could be developed to either take the resident to a quiet area when the roommate's visitors were present or to request that the roommate take visitors to the lounge. Likewise, if the resident becomes paranoid (suspicious) at night because her impaired vision causes her to view shadows as people hiding in her room, room lighting could be adjusted to prevent shadows from being cast.

Let's review some of the behavioral problems that residents may display and some ways you can help the situation.

Aggressiveness:
- Can include hitting, kicking, biting, threatening, falsely accusing, insulting
- Possible causes/contributing factors: dementia, paranoia, anxiety, anger, feelings of powerlessness
- Measures to help:
  - Know situations that promote aggressive behaviors and avoid them if possible

71

- Identify and note signs that can warn you that the behavior is going to take place
- Get help to protect yourself and others
- Distract the resident, relocate the resident to an area where there aren't other people
- Ignore insults and unkind comments made to you
- Allow the resident as much decision-making and control over activities as possible
- Recognize and reward positive behaviors

Wandering:
- Possible causes/contributing factors: dementia, delirium, boredom, anxiety, excess sleep, insufficient exercise, medication, side effects, misinterpretation of environment
- Measures to help:
  - Arrange for supervised walks of resident at regularly scheduled times
  - Provide activities that can help resident expend energy
  - Assure safety of environment (e.g., secured window screens, alarmed doors)
  - Check frequently on location and status of resident
  - Make sure residents wear ID bracelet at all times, keep recent photo of resident in record
  - Offer toileting assistance at regular intervals
  - Orient resident to environment and reorient as needed
  - Keep areas in which resident could wander well-lighted

Signs of Medical Emergencies

Pulmonary Embolism
Shortness of breath
Increased respirations
Chest discomfort
ECG and x-ray changes
Low blood oxygen
Dyspnea and hemoptysis
  may/may not be present
Tachycardia may be absent
  if resident taking beta
  blocker or has disease of
  cardiac conduction

Myocardial Infarction
Confusion
Sudden dyspnea
Weakness
Pain radiating to arm,
  chest, neck, abdomen
  (although pain is not
  always present)
Moist, pale skin
Decreased blood pressure
Low grade fever
Elevated sedimentation rate

Angina
Mild->severe pain at
  middle to upper portion
  of sternum, radiating to
  neck, jaws, sternum
Tight, vice-like feeling
  around chest
Weakness
Numbness in arms, hands
Apprehension

Pneumonia
Confusion
Increased respirations
Dehydration
Fatigue
Anorexia
Cough (may be non-
  productive)
Fever (may not be of a
  high spiking nature)
Chest pain (may be absent)
Abnormal breath sounds
Elevated WBC may not
  be present

Congestive Heart Failure
Dyspnea at rest
Shortness of breath
Fatigue
Confusion
Rapid weight gain
Left-sided failure: cough,
  orthopnea, dyspnea on
  exertion, nocturia,
  abnormal breath sounds
Right-sided failure:
  distended neck veins,
  peripheral edema, liver
  enlargement and
  tenderness, abdominal
  distension, ascites,
  GI discomfort

continued

Signs of Medical Emergencies continued

Transient Ischemic Attack
Signs last minutes to hours
Confusion
Dizziness
Aphasia
Falling
Personality changes
Diplopia
Hemiparesis
Amnesia
Motor weakness
Unilateral loss of vision
Ataxia
Headaches

Acute Glaucoma
Severe pain in/around eye
Nausea, vomiting
Blurred vision
Perception of seeing halos
  around lights

Detached Retina
Sudden or gradual onset
  of symptoms
Blurred vision
Blank areas—>complete
  loss of vision
Puffy face
Absence of sweating
Feeling of coating over eye

Hyperthermia
Confusion
Rectal temperature >102° F
Rapid, weak pulse
Weakness
Headache
Hot, dry skin
Nausea, vomiting
Muscle cramps
Loss of consciousness

Hypothermia
Confusion
Decreased level of
  consciousness
Rectal temperature <95°F
Decreased pulse
Slower respirations
Gray skin color
Cold skin
Puffy face
Absence of sweating

Inappropriate Sexual Behavior
- Can include exposing self, touching others, masturbation in view of others
- Possible causes/contributing factors include: dementia, misinterpretation of actions of others (e.g., thinking that an innocent hug is a sexual advance), loss of inhibition from disease or medications, increase ed libido due to medications (e.g., L-dopa), itching or discomfort of genitalia
- Measures to help:
  - Inform resident that behavior is inappropriate
  - Relocate resident to private area
  - Distract resident with other activities
  - Provide acceptable forms of touch (e.g., stroking pet, holding hand)
  - Assure staff are not giving messages that could be misinterpreted (e.g., wearing tight pants or clothing that exposes cleavage, playfully flirting)
  - Ask resident about need for toileting

Emergencies

LTCF residents can experience the same acute problems as any other adult. You need to identify symptoms that could be due to emergency conditions and assure that these are communicated to the physician or nurse practitioner as soon as possible. When reporting changes in status such as these, be sure to describe the symptoms, general condition of the resident, current vital signs, results of recent lab tests, and recent medications and treatments that were given. On the page that follow are signs of some emergency conditions that you may encounter.

Chapter 4

SAFE MEDICATION ADMINISTRATION

Medication administration is a major responsibility of LPNs in LTCFs. It also is one that is quite challenging in terms of the huge amount of information you must know in order to administer drugs safely. Let's look at some of the issues.

Many, Many Drugs

One of the challenges of drug use in residents has to do with polypharmacy–the large number of drugs consumed. On the average, each nursing home resident receives six different drugs daily and it is not unusual to find residents who receive a dozen different drugs each day.

As the number of drugs used increases, so does the risk of drug-drug interactions. Drugs can interact with each other and produce:

Synergistic effects: when given together, some drugs can increase the effects of each other (e.g., antidepressants could increase the effects of antianxiety drugs, anti-inflammatory drugs could increase the effects of anticoagulants)

Antagonistic effects: the effects of some drugs can be reduced when given with certain other drugs (e.g., antacids can decrease the effects of digitalis and antipsychotic drugs)

Drugs also can interact with food. For example, a lot of caffeine intake can reduce the effectiveness of colchicine and probenecid. A high intake of alkaline foods (e.g., milk, cream, almonds) can prolong the action of some antihistamines. A high protein diet can reduce the effectiveness of levodopa. It is useful to have the pharmacist and nutritionist review the medications residents are taking for possible drug-food interactions.

Effects of Age-Related Changes

The advanced age of many residents contributes to additional problems with medication use. Age-related changes impact the body's ability to absorb, metabolize and excrete drugs. For instance:

- Absorption can be impaired due to decreases in gastric acid, absorptive surface, and gastrointestinal motility
- Reduced circulation to the vagina and lower bowel slow the melting of suppositories
- Decreased body fluids can lead to high concentrations of water-soluble substances (e.g., vitamins B1, B2, B6 and C)
- Increased proportion of fat tissue in older bodies can cause the accumulation of fat-soluble drugs (e.g., barbiturates, diazepam, and lidocaine) to toxic levels
- Reduced albumin concentration can alter the distribution of protein-bound drugs (e.g., phenytoin, phenylbutazone, warfain)
- Less effective metabolism of drugs can result from decreases in liver blood flow and enzyme activity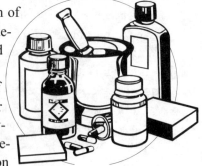
- Delayed excretion of drugs (leading to their accumulation to toxic levels) can be caused by reductions in kidney function

78

These changes demand differences in prescribing patterns (most drugs should be prescribed at lower dosages for older residents) and close observation of the effectiveness of and reactions to drug therapy.

Psychotropic Drugs

A particular area of concern is the use of psychotropic drugs in residents. Psychotropics are drugs that affect the mind, such as antipsychotics (major tranquilizers), antianxiety/hypnotic drugs, and antidepressants. Studies indicate that 35% to 65% of nursing home residents are receiving some type of psychotropic drug. Although these drugs can enhance he quality of life for residents and enable them to be more functional, these drugs also carry the risk for profound adverse reactions.

Psychotropic drugs are considered a form of *chemical* restraints so they need to be used only when absolutely necessary. Never should they be used for the convenience of staff.

Regulations state that:
- each resident's drug regimen be free from unnecessary drugs
- antipsychotic drugs be administered only to treat specific conditions as documented in the resident's record and following a comprehensive assessment
- once administered, antipsychotic drugs be gradually reduced in dosage in an attempt to discontinue the drug unless there is a contraindication for doing so

---

If psychotropic drugs are used, the following guidelines are helpful to follow:
- Use psychotropic drugs only when other measures are ineffective and only for the management of specific targeted behaviors
- Begin with the smallest possible dosage and gradually increase, if necessary, to achieve desired results
- Monitor and document administration, effectiveness, and

side effects. Be specific about the effects on the resident's behavior
- Assure an adequate time of administration has been provided to achieve results, recognizing that several weeks of therapy may be required before effectiveness is noted
- Ask about drug holidays to minimize the cumulative (build up) effects of the drug (Drug holidays are days when the drug is not given---in other words, a "day off" from the drug)
- Use behavioral interventions and other therapeutic approaches to supplement the drug

The high risk for serious adverse drug reactions in residents demands that drugs be used with discretion and caution. Granted, the physician prescribes the medication, but in reality, the information and request communicated to the physician by nursing often determines if a drug is prescribed or not. Advise your nursing staff that they best advocate for residents when they attempt to address a symptom with an option other than a drug, if at all possible. For example, if a resident is agitated, taking him for a short walk or massaging his shoulders while speaking calmly to him may bring about a change in his behavior without the need for a tranquilizer. Likewise, rather than requesting a laxative, staff can offer the resident juices and foods known to stimulate a bowel movement for her. *You* can affect the number and type of drugs that are ordered for a resident.

The following pages outlines measures that you can take to assure you are helping residents to use medications safely.

Measures to Promote
Safe Medication Use

- Know the medications you are administering. If you are giving a drug that you're not familiar with, look it up first.

- Understand the intended purposes for the drugs you are giving to a resident so that you can assess their effectiveness

- Whenever possible, use measures other than drugs to manage problems (e.g., dietary changes rather than a laxative, backrub rather than a sedative)

- Make sure PRN orders clearly state the conditions for which the drugs are to be used and that you administer them for these conditions

- Check that drugs have been ordered in correct dosages. If you believe the dosage is incorrect, discuss this with you supervisor or the physician before you administer the drug.

- Explain to residents the purposes of their drugs

- Make sure you are administering the correct drug, to the correct resident, at the correct time

- Know the adverse effects of all drugs you give

- Report any possible adverse effects promptly

- Make sure the blood pressures are checked at least weekly for residents taking antihypertensive drugs

- Check residents who are receiving anticoagulant drugs for signs of bleeding; make sure their prothrombin time has been checked at least monthly or as ordered

continued...

Measures to Promote
Safe Medication Use
(continued)

- Check the pulse of residents who use cardiovascular drugs

- Make sure that blood glucose is checked at least every 60 days or as ordered for residents taking hypoglycemic drugs

- Know the stop order date for antibiotics that you administer

- Assure residents who are taking diuretics have serum potassium levels evaluated regularly, as ordered

- If intravenous (IV) therapy is used, monitor carefully and identify and report complications, such as infiltration, redness

- Regularly review all medications residents receive for their effectiveness and to be sure the benefits outweigh the side effects

- Keep the medication cart and compartments locked when unattended

- Check for changes in drug orders before administering drugs

- Record the drugs you administer as soon as you give them

- Document omitted drugs, along with the reason for their omission

- Report and record medication errors according to your facility's procedure

Chapter 5

MANAGEMENT ASPECTS

Nurse Williams begins the shift by listening to report, reviewing the records of residents for which she is responsible, and thinking through the needs that these residents can be expected to have during the next 8 hours. She notes the staff who are on duty and assigns them responsibilities on the basis of their competencies. On reviewing new orders, she identifies the need for medications and supplies and calls in requests to the appropriate departments. Throughout the shift she checks on the care staff is giving, and corrects and guides staff when their services aren't meeting acceptable standards. When residents have symptoms or new problems, she communicates this to the assistant director of nursing who then communicates this information to the physician. She stops to respond to visitors' questions and to assist as needed. At the completion of the shift Nurse Williams gets report from each of the staff on her team and documents accordingly. She ends her shift by doing rounds and giving report to the nurse coming on duty.

Perhaps you can relate to Nurse Williams because you have been assigned certain management functions. These management activities often become so routine that you may do them automatically without much thought. However, these seemingly minor activities involve management functions that are based on complex processes. Consider that Nurse Williams' activities required that she:

- Have knowledge of the usual operations of the unit and the facility's policies and procedures
- Be familiar with the competencies and work style of each employee on her team
- Know the amount of time and supplies/equipment required for each residents' care
- Match the residents' caregiving needs to the available resources
- Be able to communicate effectively within the nursing department and with other departments
- Respond to unplanned events and solve problems
- Use observational and interview skills to evaluate the care being given
- Coach, guide, and educate staff in proper techniques
- Monitor unit activities
- Determine if tasks have been done at the end of the shift

The planning, organizing, leading, and monitoring activities described above fall within the area of management functions.

Skills That You'll Need

Being a great bedside nurse doesn't make someone a good manager. Being given the title of "charge nurse" or "team leader" doesn't automatically cause someone to be a good manager. There are certain skills that are needed if you're going to be a manager; let's take a look at some of the major ones.

Assertiveness

A team leader learns that one of the nursing assistants has called in and reassigns the absent employee's residents to the other CNAs. Upon looking at the revised assignment sheet,

84

CNA Cumo says "I have enough to do with my regular caseload and I don't plan to take on any more work." This starts the other CNAs grumbling and complaining about their assignments. The team leader nervously says, "Well, all right. Don't worry. I'll do the assignment myself."

Charge nurse Carter approaches CNA Green and tells him to go to the supply room for some room deodorant. Mr. Green begins to reply, "But Mrs. Carter, I'm right in the middle of..." when Mrs. Carter interrupts him and shouts, "I don't care what you're doing and I don't expect any lip from you when I give you an order. Just drop what you're doing and do what I tell you!"

These are two examples of the extremes of nonassertive behavior. In the first example, the team leader has the right and responsibility to reassign an absent employee's caseload; but, pressure from the CNAs caused the team leader to back away from her responsibility and take the entire caseload on herself. There is a strong probability that the team leader will be overworked and some of her responsibilities will be done less than perfectly. In the second example, Mrs. Carter had the right to request Mr. Green to go to the supply room, but she also had a responsibility to hear his response and not to be so aggressive toward him. Mr. Green may have been in the middle of an important caregiving activity that he couldn't drop without jeopardizing the safety of a resident, but he never got the chance to explain that. He is put in a no-win situation in which he either risks harming a resident by leaving in the middle of a task or risks harming his work record by disobeying his supervisor.

Now that you've seen examples of what assertiveness isn't, let's look at what assertiveness *is*.

Assertive behavior involves the protection of your legitimate rights. Whether it is refusing to allow someone else to make an important decision for you or asking someone to avoid blowing smoke in your face, you have the right to protect what is yours, to exercise control over your own life, and to avoid unpleasant situations. As a manager, you have the right to make reasonable requests of the CNAs you supervise without feeling badly or having to apologize.

The protection of your rights isn't at the expense of another person's rights if done assertively. Ideally, there is no winner or loser when you defend your rights. Just as no one has a right to make us feel uncomfortable, threatened, frustrated, or imposed upon, we have no right to create those feelings in others. An assertive interaction allows both parties to feel good and safe.

Assertiveness is displayed through speech and behavior. Fumbling for words or speaking in a meek manner does not convey assertiveness. Likewise, blushing, nervously twitching, and avoiding eye contact reflects nonassertiveness, regardless of what words are spoken.

There is nothing tricky or complex about behaving assertively. In fact, the key to assertiveness is basic, direct honesty. Long explanations or apologies are unnecessary. For instance, you don't have to go into a long story about how you have a history of asthma in order to get someone to stop smoking in your face. Instead, it is enough to say, "I'd appreciate if you would not blow smoke in my face." Simple and to the point will do.

It can be useful for you to consider how assertive you are. Answer the questions that follow to help gain insight into your behavior.

Are You Assertive?

Answer the following questions with yes or no:

- Are you reluctant to speak up and state your opinion?
- Do you do what others tell you to do, even when you don't believe it is correct or you don't want to?
- Do you find it difficult to express positive and negative feelings to others?
- If someone is behaving in a manner that disturbs you, do you allow it to continue rather than confront the person?
- Do you allow others to make your decisions, or do you make decisions for other people that they should be making on their own?
- To avoid disappointing others, do you say yes when you really want to say no?
- Do you intimidate or bully others in order to get your way, or do you allow yourself to be intimidated by others?
- Is it difficult for you to discontinue an interaction with a salesperson when you really do not want the product?
- Are you hesitant to introduce yourself to a new person?
- When you feel you have been taken advantage of or not treated fairly, do you stew inside but not express yourself openly?
- Do you find it hard to give or accept compliments or criticisms?

If you've answered *yes* to many of these questions, you may need to beef up your assertiveness skills. It is useful to try to identify the specific areas that are problems for you. For example, you may behave assertively at work, but allow your spouse to take advantage of you. Or, you may be able to defend your rights to a salesperson, but permit your supervisor to treat you unfairly. Once you've identified where your problems are, you can address and correct them.

Practice helps to increase your assertiveness skills. Begin practicing with people who are close to you and with whom a secure relationship exists. After gaining some confidence and skill, broaden your scope. You also can practice mentally, by rehearsing the situation in your mind before actually confronting it. For example, if you're going to meet with your supervisor to discuss a promotion, think what the conversation will be. What type of reaction will your supervisor have, what type of questions will be raised? Think through as many consequences as possible and prepare assertive reactions for each.

It's also helpful to find good role models and watch them in action. Analyze their behaviors and try to determine what makes them effective. If possible, ask these individuals for advice and feedback.

As a nurse manager, you have a responsibility for helping others become assertive, too. Some of the staff you work with may come from backgrounds in which aggressive behavior is the norm; some may believe that people must be passive with their superiors and not express views. Teach others about assertiveness and encourage them to communicate assertively. When nonassertive behaviors are demonstrated, tactfully bring them to the person's attention and offer suggestions on ways that the person can behave more assertively.

Communication

Communication is the thread that holds all operations of a facility together. Consider some of the essential communications that occur in a routine day on the nursing unit. The unit nurse manager is informed of the number of staff that will be on duty for the day, the intershift report gives information on the current status of residents, the care plan presents the unique care needs for each resident, staff request necessary supplies, residents voice needs, policies are announced, staff share their changes about residents, records show residents' current status, families telephone for information, meal changes are sent to the dietary department–and the list goes on. Often many different types of communication are involved in basic activities (just consider all the verbal and written communication that occurs with a new admission). Stop communication and the facility's operations become dysfunctional.

The fact that many types of communication occur in the course of a routine day does not mean that communications are necessarily effective. Communication is a complex process with many areas for potential breakdown. The basic process of communication is as follows:

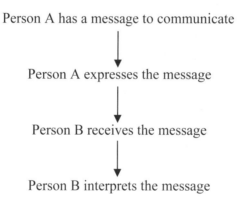

Person A has a message to communicate

Person A expresses the message

Person B receives the message

Person B interprets the message

The process seems simple until all the variables the could impact it are considered, such as the communication skills of each person, the relationship between the individuals, environmental interferences, and the mode of expression. Consider the following examples:

*The nurse manager wants to communicate dissatisfaction
to the director of nursing for denying the request
for reimbursement to attend a workshop*

↓

*The nurse manager writes a memo to the DON stating,
"I understand your reasons for denying my request and
hope this type of request can be approved in the future."*

↓

*The DON reads the memo and becomes suspicious of the rea-
son the nurse manager wrote a memo rather than discussing
the   issue. The DON believes the nurse manager is trying to
build documentation to use against the DON.*

In this example, the form of communication that the nurse manager selected–memo–put the DON on the defensive. The DON
was more concerned about the use of a memo than the sub-
stance of the communication.

Let's look at another example:

*The nurse manager appreciates that although the new
CNA was carrying an extra caseload, he completed
his entire assignment well*

↓

*The nurse manager says to the CNA, "I'm surprised
that you were able to do all that work."*

↓

*The CNA hears the comment and interprets it to mean that the
nurse manager didn't think he was competent enough to do the
work and surprised to learn that he is*

Here, the nurse manager gave an indirect compliment, which perhaps may have been her style. However, the new CNA isn't familiar with the fact that this was the way the nurse manager gave a compliment, misinterpreted her intent, and was offended. You see how even the simplest communication can create major headaches.

If communication between two people appears complicated, imagine the problems that can arise when communication travels through several people. If you've ever played the game where a whispered comment was passed through a group, only to have the last person hear something that wasn't anywhere near the original comment, you may understand the risk for communication breakdown when you increase the people involved. Unfortunately, in the average facility, information must be communicated through several layers of staff. And, like the whispered comment game, the message the last recipient of the information receives, may bear no resemblance to the original one. This can create serious problems in that staff may be uninformed or misinformed of policies and procedures, feel insecure because they lack information about what is happening in the facility, and receive messages with the content or tone different from what was originally intended. Communication breakdowns are real and frequent in any organization, but they can be reduced. Some hints for improving communication are offered below.

Hints to Improving Communication

- *Be clear on what you want to express.* Think through the purpose and content of the communication before sending the message. Weigh the risks and gains associated with the communication.

- *Select the best means of communicating the message.* Verbal communication may be more personal and faster in some situations, whereas written communication provides a record for future reference and ensures that all people receive the same message. At times, an informal grapevine can be valuable in spreading information rapidly when official communication is undesired or impossible.

- *Keep a healthy balance of communication.* Insufficient communication can cause staff to feel uncertain of expectations, policies, and operations. They may make mistakes because they are misinformed or feel that they're not considered important because information isn't shared with them. At the other extreme, too much communication can result in information overload. Staff may receive many memos and announcements that they tune them out. Employees need enough information to perform their work and remain current of facility operations without being overburdened.

- *Keep communication as simple and direct as possible.* Express the message in as few words as possible. The purpose of the communication isn't to show how many fancy words you know but to deliver a message. Complicated words and phrases can be difficult for some employees to understand and cause confusion. Effective communication uses as few words as possible and sends a clear message.

- *Use examples to enhance understanding.* For instance, rather than writing a memo that says, "Any employee having indications of infection should report to the infection control nurse," it would be more useful to say, "Any employee with a fever, diarrhea, vomiting, skin rash, sore

Table 8-1 Self Assessment of Time Wasters

How often do I:	Often	Some-times	Rarely
Start the day with no agenda/plan?		✓	
Feel prioritizing and making lists are a waste of time?			✓
Address problems as they confront me rather than by priority?		✓	
Answer most incoming telephone calls myself?	✓		
Try to do several tasks at one time?	✓		
Allow unscheduled visitors and calls to interrupt me?		✓	
Feel uncomfortable delegating tasks?		✓	
Find it easier to do things myself rather than ask others?		✓	
Feel it is inappropriate to close my door and limit interruptions?		✓	
Require my approval for staff's direct care actions?			✓
Require most decisions funnel through me?			✓
Feel subordinates are unwilling to accept responsibility?	✓		✓
Feel uneasy if a subordinate does a job better than I?		✓	
Feel it is impossible to take a day off?		✓	
Insist of perfection	✓		
Column subtotal	4	8	il

93

Table 8-1 Self Assessment of Time Wasters (continued)

How often do I:	Often	Some-times	Rarely
Postpone projects until all conditions are perfect?			`
Procrastinate?	´		
Conduct meetings without an agenda?		´	
Attend meetings that lack an agenda?		`	
Feel reluctant to make decisions without staff discussion?	´		
Listen to staff's personal problems?	`		
Discuss my personal life at work?	-		
Postpone attending to my symptoms?	\		
Make mistakes or get distracted due to poorly managed stress?		`	
Fail to engage in self-care practices?	`		
Column subtotal	4	3	1
Column subtotal from previous page	4	4	4
Combined columns total	10	11	5
Multiply	**X 4**	**X 3**	**X 2**
Column score	40	33	10

Add all 3 column scores together
A score **under 60** means you're probably doing a good job managing your time. Congratulations!
A score of **60-75** means you could stand to make some changes and improve your time management.
A score **above 75** implies you need to pay major attention to improving your time management

throat, boil, cold symptoms, or any other sign of infection should report to the infection control nurse."

- *Always match actions with the communication.* If you have told CNAs that you are starting a new way of giving out assignments on Monday, you should be ready to do so on Monday. Your communication will have little credibility if you do not do what you say.
- *Keep the layers between you and the recipient of your communication as few as possible.* Each additional receiver and sender in the communication process increases the risk of miscommunication. If a message is important, try to tell the people involved directly.
- *Follow up to assure people got the message.* Making an announcement or sending a memo is no guarantee that people will do what is expected. Use spot checks, observe, and have informal conversations to evaluate how well the message was received and understood.
- *Recognize that listening is a crucial part of communication.* It is important to pay careful attention to what is being communicated to you. Frequently, people become so involved thinking about their response that they miss what is being said. Effective communication requires that you learn to discipline yourself to hear and understand the other person. Full attention, eye contact, nodding responses, and acknowledgement of what the other person has said are ways of being a good listener.

Time Management

Learning to manage your time is a very important skill, not only to your role as nurse manager, but in other roles in your life in general. The reality is that your list of things to do will grow while the amount of time in a day stays the same. So, unless you have a secret for extending your day to 30 hours, you'll find it useful to be a good manager of your time.

The fact that you are busy and putting in long hours doesn't mean that you really *need* to be chronically busy and working more hours than everyone else. Time can be spent in activities that are inappropriate or unnecessary for you to do, or that are nonproductive. To get a sense of how this affects you, complete the self-assessment on the pages that follow.

If your score indicates that you have some time wasting behaviors to correct, take a look at the type of behaviors that trip you up the most. Common time wasting behaviors include:

Inefficient work style: starting the day without a plan, allowing unnecessary interruptions, failing to complete one task before getting involved in another, procrastinating

Excessive control: unwillingness to delegate tasks that can be performed by others, getting involved with caregiving tasks of CNAs

Unnecessary and ineffective meetings: conducting meetings without an agenda and time limit, having regularly scheduled meetings regardless of need, allowing team members to divert meeting to non-agenda items, conducting meetings when the same outcomes could be achieved through email, memo, or other means

Unnecessary perfectionism: insisting that there be 100% perfection when it isn't essential, holding to unrealistically high standards

Personal problems: frequently discussing personal problems or activities, getting involved in the personal lives of staff, allowing nonemergency telephone calls during work hours, feeling a need to prove worth by working longer or harder than others

Poor self-care habits: failing to be assertive in setting limits, obtaining insufficient sleep and rest, ineffectively managing stress, feeling chronically fatigued due to poor diet or insufficient exercise, postponing attention to personal health conditions or symptoms

Keeping a time log for several days also assists you in identifying specific time wasting behaviors. A log can help you to identify patterns, such as the same few people interrupting you or schedule-disrupting crises that resulted because you didn't take the time to plan for a situation.

A review of the way you use time and a self-assessment of time wasters can aid you in identifying specific practices that need to be changed to promote an improved use of time. Some strategies to improve time management could include:

- **Plan:** Determine tasks that need to be accomplished and plot them on a calendar (e.g., activities to be done over the next year, month, week). Be sure to set realistic time frames and accept only those responsibilities that can be achieved within the real limitations that exist. Monitor progress against the scheduled plans.
- **Prioritize:** Rank tasks according to priority for accomplishment, e.g.:
    A= top priority, must be done as soon as possible
    B= can wait until later date without significant consequences
    C= nonessential
- **Recognize the difference between important and urgent**. An important task needs to be accomplished but can wait (e.g., routine review of the charts), while an urgent task must be done as soon as possible (e.g., calling the doctor with a resident's abnormal lab report).
- **Act in a timely manner:** Try to respond to emails and other correspondence when they are read to avoid re-reading and additional handling. Return calls as soon as a convenient time is available. Postponing activities can lead to time be-

ing wasted in having to refresh your memory at a later time and only will increase the accumulated workload.

- **Delegate:** Delegate tasks that can be and are supposed to be done by the others on your team. Delegation also affords staff the opportunity to develop skills and grow in their jobs.
- **Work smarter:** Putting in long hours does not equate to being effective. There certainly will be times when you'll have to work overtime, but if this is a regular occurrence, explore the reason (e.g., unrealistic demands, insufficient staff, unrealistically high expectations, inefficient work style, lack of competency, poor personal health, distractions, etc.) and develop strategies to correct or improve them.
- **Practice good self-care:** Learn to protect your time and set limits. Only participate on committees and in activities that are productive; try to withdraw from those that are not. Refuse to allow others to abuse your time. Make time for leisure and the things that are truly important to you and your well-being. Balance work with ample leisure and "down time" so that you remain healthy. You may find it useful to block out "Personal Time" on your calendar and honor it as you would any important appointment.

Delegation

Delegation refers to the transfer of responsibility and authority for an activity to another person. When you are given management responsibilities, such as leading a team, you will have certain responsibilities delegated to you and you will be expected to delegate tasks to others.

It is important that you only accept responsibilities that you are allowed to do by law, as stated in your Nurse Practice Act. If you don't have a copy of your state's Nurse Practice Act for LPNs contact your state board of nursing and get one. Likewise, you should not delegate responsibilities to others that they are not allowed to do by law. For example, if a CNA is not allowed to administer medications, you cannot instruct the CNA to do so, even if you feel confident that the CNA could handle this with no problem. The moral of the story: *know the regulations governing the employees you supervise and be sure to only give them tasks that they are allowed to perform.* Inappropriate delegation can get you and the person to whom you delegated in a heap of trouble.

When you delegate a task, you still are accountable. For example, if you have six CNAs on your team and assign them each the care of a caseload of residents, you cannot assume that because they are trained and able to give the assigned care, that it will be given. The following guidelines can help you delegate responsibly.

Guidelines for Delegation

- Know the guidelines for delegation established by your state's Nurse Practice Act and your facility's policies.
- Be clear on the task that is to be accomplished.
- Know the time and resources required for the task.
- Make sure the employee has the competencies and capabilities to do the task.
- Clarify the level of delegation that is needed:
  - delegation of the task without additional follow-up (e.g., telling a CNA to take a resident to the bathroom without having the CNA report back to you)
  - delegation with periodic progress checks (e.g., assigning a new CNA a resident and checking on the care being given every half hour)
  - delegation with review and approval of each step toward completion (e.g., assigning a new CNA a resident and asking that the CNA call you before she gets the resident out of bed, feeds

99

the resident, measures I/O)
- Give the assignment in a clear and complete manner
  - describe the responsibilities and time frame to complete them
  - state the goal and priorities
  - describe landmarks/steps in reaching the goal
  - encourage the employee to seek clarification if needed
  - make sure that the task is understood
  - assure the employee has the time and capability to do the job
- Periodically check the progress and obtain feedback
- Give feedback; offer praise for a job well done

Monitoring Performance

As mentioned, when you delegate a task, you need to check on the progress and determine if it is being done properly. There are a variety of methods that you can use to monitor the performance of staff for whom you are responsible:

        direct observation
        periodic checks; spot checks
        verbal feedback from employees
        interviews with residents and visitors
        consulting with staff
        absenteeism records
        incident and accident reports
        reports of quality assurance assessments

As you make rounds on units, you can find it beneficial to carry index cards or a pocket-sized notebook to record observations. These anecdotal notes should include both positive and negative findings, action taken (if any), residents or employees involved, date, and time; at the end of the shift you can store these notes in your personal files or share them with your supervisor. Patterns of performance problems can be detected through a periodic review of these notations. The factual data contained on anecdotal notes can prove valuable in supporting comments on evaluations and in assuring that the evaluation reflect overall performance and not merely the most recent event that can be recalled. Of course, serious problems shouldn't wait until an annual evaluation to be addressed. The object is not to accumulate evidence for a poor evaluation, but instead, to identify performance problems in need of improvement.

"Problem Behaviors"

The term "problem employee" sometimes is used to describe an individual who has a behavior, personality, or characteristic displayed in the workplace that is disruptive, annoying, or otherwise a problem. In reality, it is the employee's behavior that is the problem and by focusing on the behavior, generalizations about the individual employee can be avoided.

Correction of the "problem behavior" begins by understanding some of the possible causes of the behavior. Once the causes are understood, specific actions can be planned to correct the behavior. Examples of some common problem behaviors include:

Complaining Some employees seem to constantly gripe and find something negative in most ideas and activities. Complaining may bring rewards to these employees in the attention they receive and the leadership they achieve by hitting a sensitive chord with dissatisfied coworkers. Complaining could indicate a refusal to assume responsibility or a feeling of powerlessness. Efforts to change this behavior could include listening and acknowledging the complainer's views without implying agreement. Try to get specific examples rather than allowing the person to make broad generalizations (e.g., "these things never work", "the administrator always takes the word of families over staff.") Ask the complainer to suggest solutions to the problems identified. Also, consider conducting a staff meeting in which staff are invited to list problems, identify problems that can be corrected, and make recommendations for correction; problems that cannot be corrected (e.g., layout of facility) should be identified and staff asked to agree to cease complaining about them. Finally, state the facts or decision without apology and move ahead.

Passive-aggressive behavior There are individuals who give all the signals of agreeing and complying on the surface, but attempt to destroy plans and actions behind your back, or act out by pouting and making others feel guilty. These behaviors can reflect the lack of assertiveness or confidence to express feelings and opinions directly, anger, or a sense of powerlessness. Passive-aggressive behavior can be changed by encouraging employees to express their opinions in a constructive manner and respecting the opinions when they are expressed. Individuals who continue this behavior after being provided channels for openly expressing their views should be confronted with their behaviors, informed that their behaviors are unacceptable, and assisted in their efforts to change.

Know-it-all Some employees are self-proclaimed experts who claim to know more than everyone else (including their supervisors) and who tend to be closed to new ideas or suggestions. Often, they are insensitive to the views of others, believing their opinions are the best and only ones. Individuals displaying this behavior may have a need for recognition or status, or may possess only a superficial understanding of the issue at hand. To effectively work with these individuals, acknowledge and show appreciation for their contribution, but communicate that you'd like to try a different approach, and invite their assistance, if possible. In some circumstances, these individuals may possess greater expertise in some areas; don't hesitate putting their expertise to constructive use and giving them the recognition they deserve.

Negativism There are employees who attempt to destroy new ideas by informing others of the many reasons "why it won't work." Persons with a negative attitude may be afraid of change, feel powerless, or perhaps, have witnessed in the past attempts to implement unrealistic or inappropriate ideas. Often, these individuals can gain the support of coworkers by playing on the little seeds of doubt and the potential for despair that may exist in others. It is useful to try to include negative people in the planning stage of a project so that they may feel some ownership, understand the idea, and be more likely to support it. It can prove useful to discuss the issue and ask for the worse case scenario to aid in diffusing negative views. If the involvement of employees who tend to be negative cannot be obtained, they should be limited in the amount of influence they can exercise over coworkers. Realistic optimism should be displayed to counterbalance the influence of negativists. Behaviors that are supportive should be recognized and rewarded.

Excuses Some employees seem to invest more effort in explaining why they haven't done or cannot do something than would be required if they just went ahead and did the task. These individuals may be trying to avoid responsibility, or may lack the skills and knowledge to perform the task. For some employees, making excuses is a means of controlling the situation when they feel powerless. It is important to avoid getting sidetracked, and to stick to the issue at hand and reinforce the expectation clearly and directly.

Silence Silence makes many people uncomfortable, and some employees use this to their advantage. During a meeting or counseling session, these employees may not respond or make any verbal contribution. In an effort to deal with uncomfortable silence, others may fill in the void with their own comments which enables the silence-keepers to escape responsibility for participation. An effective means of changing this behavior is to resist the temptation to fill in the silence and remain silent until the employee responds. If 5-10 minutes pass without comment, reschedule a time to meet and inform the silence-keepers that they will be given additional time to get their thoughts together; schedule several sessions if necessary.

Underachieving Some employees have the potential to perform at much higher levels than they actually demonstrate. The reasons for their underachievement could include their being in a job that is not challenging for them or the lack of motivators. Underachievers should be evaluated to determine the match of their capabilities to the demands of the job; job expansion or assistance in climbing the career ladder should be offered, if indicated. If low motivation is the cause, determine the motivational needs that are not being met and attempt to supply this motivations (e.g., opportunity to demonstrate new skill, recognition of good work, reinforcing security of job), if possible.

There are many reasons, often complex ones, for behaviors that cause problems in the workplace. These behaviors may follow a long pattern that has been established and practiced within one's family or culture. The personalities of some individuals contribute to certain behavioral patterns. The behaviors, although a problem in the workplace, may bring rewards to the employees demonstrating them. Also, some employees may be unaware of expected or appropriate workplace behavior, and unknowingly may be behaving in unacceptable ways.

People can change their behaviors and some measures that

can assist them in doing so are described on the next page. An important responsibility that you have as you wear the manager hat is to help employees develop positive behaviors by teaching, coaching, counseling, encouraging, and role-modeling. Rewarding positive behaviors and helping employees to achieve high levels of performance are consistent with that responsibility.

Measures to Assist An Employee in Changing Negative Behaviors

- describe to the employee the behavior and its impact
- clearly define the acceptable behavior that should be substituted
- invite suggestions from the employee as to how he or she can be helped to change
- hold the employee accountable
- recognize and reward positive/acceptable behaviors
- model desired behaviors yourself

Managing Complaints

When you accept management responsibilities, part of what you can expect is to be the recipient of complaints. In fact, complaints are not a rare occurrence which probably comes as little surprise. Being dependent on staff and not having good health, residents may be impatient of staff. Families may express their guilt, anger and frustration over having to institutionalize a loved one through criticisms of staff. Residents and families may have unrealistic expectations. In addition, many real problems may occur, such as the loss of residents' personal property, delays in responding to requests, and poor staff attitudes. These situations create fertile territory for complaints.

Most individuals understand that problems and misunderstandings can occur in a complex organization, such as a long-term care facility. Although people may not be pleased with problem situations, they usually are willing to be understanding and forgiving if they feel they are treated fairly. On the other hand, a lack of sensitivity to their complaints and defensive attitude from staff can cause minor problems to snowball into major ones, and lead to dissatisfied individuals seeking legal recourse to resolve problems.

Actively Prevent Complaints

Ideally, complaint management begins with *complaint prevention*. Staff should be aware of the types of problems that result in the most complaints and work to avoid having them occur. For instance, if staff identify that many complaints arise when visitors find their relatives wet or still in bed at the start of visiting hours, staff should schedule their work to assure that residents can be changed and gotten out of bed prior to the start of visiting hours. Likewise, if residents complain that their clothing is not returned from the laundry, staff should make an effort to check that all clothing is clearly labeled with the residents' names before being put in the linen hamper. Often, complaints arise from small problems that can be corrected.

Prepare Residents and Families

Preparing residents and families for the realities of nursing home care also can reduce complaints. Ideally, families and residents should receive an orientation to the facility's operations that describes normal routines, services that are provided and services that cannot be provided. For example, it may be helpful for families to understand that a tub bath will be given twice a week rather than daily, not because the staff is lazy, but because this is helpful to older skin. Likewise, informing families and residents of the hazards of immobility can aid them in

106

understanding why staff may encourage residents to get out of bed on days that they may rather not. Be honest about services that cannot be expected; for instance, families and residents need to understand that staff most likely will not be able to provide regular manicures, walk residents outdoors for one-half hour each day, or hand wash residents' nightgowns.

Welcome Feedback

Tell residents and families that the facility is interested in hearing about problems, and tell them the proper mechanism for voicing complaints. Not only will this demonstrate to residents and families the facility's interest in helping them resolve problems, but it could help the facility identify and correct situations that could potentially lead to litigation.

The facility must post for residents and visitors the process for filing complaints with the state licensing agency. Staff should not interfere with residents' right to voice complaints to outside agencies.

All staff should gain skill in managing complaints. An outline of points to remember in complaint management is offered on the next page.

Management involves many important functions. As a manager you'll be able to:

- influence care
- contribute to the development of employees
- increase your own skills.

However, responsibilities for other employees also increase your risks as you can be liable for some of the activities performed by the staff you manage. You can protect yourself and your facility by:

- staying within your Nurse Practice Act and job description
- following policies and procedures carefully
- assuring the tasks you delegate are performed well
- knowing your limitations

Hints for Managing Complaints

- Listen carefully to the full complaint. Do not interrupt or become defensive.

- Do not react to emotionally charged comments or personal criticisms of you or other staff. Try to focus the person making the complaint on the issue.

- Ask questions to obtain all the information and clarify issues. (What time did you find your husband wet? Who was the nurse who you said refused to help you?)

- Acknowledge the person's feelings without making conclusions or placing blame. (I can understand that you would be upset to find your husband in wet clothing; It is frustrating to ask for help and not get it)

- Offer to help, even if you are not the responsible party. (Let me get some dry linens and I'll change your husband now.)

- Refer the complaint to the appropriate person, following the proper channel of communication

- Inform your supervisor of the complaint.

- If tempers are flaring or the situation is getting out of control, seek the assistance of your supervisor.

- Follow-up to assure the problem has been resolved.

Chapter 6

LEGAL ASPECTS OF PRACTICE

A resident complains of fatigue and heaviness in the chest and is found to have a nonproductive cough and increased pulse rate. The unit nurse places a call to the attending physician and is unable to reach him. Over the next three hours the resident's symptoms continue and the nurse leaves additional messages for the physician. Finally, the physician returns the call and says that he will examine the resident when he visits tomorrow. The nurse tells that physician that she really thinks the resident should be examined this evening, but the physician snaps back, "Look, I've got several residents who are showing symptoms of the flu and this is just another one of them. My seeing the resident in the morning isn't going to make any difference." Reluctantly, the nurse accepts the physician's decision.

During the next shift, the resident is found dead. Autopsy reveals the cause of death to be a myocardial infarction. The unit nurse is sued for negligence for not recognizing the severity of the condition and intervening on behalf of the resident by transferring the resident to a hospital for evaluation.

It is an unusually busy day on the unit and staffing is short. Staff are running from one crisis to another and trying their best to see that everyone gets their meals and treatments. Half-way through the shift a nursing assistant reports that she is un-

able to find Mr. Hanks, a resident who has Alzheimer's disease. Staff search the entire facility but Mr. Hanks is nowhere to be found.

The facility then receives a call from the local police. Mr. Hanks was struck by a car while trying to cross a dark road. He has sustained multiple injuries and subsequently loses a leg.

Mr. Hanks' family, on behalf of the resident, sues the facility for negligence. One of the strongest argument's supporting the claim is that Mr. Hanks' care plan stated "Resident tries to leave building and requires close supervision at all times."

The unit nurse notices that CNA Clark is staggering and slurring his words. When the nurse approaches Mr. Clark she detects a strong odor of alcohol. "You need to leave the unit immediately," the nurse tells Mr. Clark. "I'm not going any-where, I'm here to work," Mr. Clark responds. Concerned that Mr. Clark will be a hazard, the nurse again orders him to leave, and again he refuses. Mr. Clark's loud tone has at-tracted the attention of other employees and visitors. "Look, Mr. Clark," the nurse says, "there is no way I am going to al-low you to work in an intoxicated condition. You need to go home and sober up." With that, the nurse takes Mr. Clark by the arm, pulls him to the lobby, and puts him in a taxi with in-structions to take him home.

Mr. Clark sues the nurse for defamation of character, as-sault, and battery.

These are examples of real situations that could occur in your own facility. A nurse doesn't want to cause trouble with a physician despite the nagging sense that the physician is not responding appropriately. Supervision and care that residents are known to need get shortchanged because there was an un-usually high rate of absenteeism on a shift. Under pressure to respond to an employee's improper behavior, the employee's rights are violated. You can see where situations like this could easily happen. None of the staff responsible for these problems intended to do any harm or commit any crime. Chances are, they are reasonably competent, caring people. But something out of the ordinary causes them to deviate from acceptable practices and the next thing they know, they are facing a lawsuit.

Growing Risks for Lawsuits in LTCFs

It's no secret that all parts of the health care system and all types of health care providers are being sued more today than ever before. LTCFs are not immune from this trend. If anything, lawsuits against LTCFs are growing and some of the reasons for this are:

Resident population: Residents of LTCFs tend to have multiple conditions that heighten their risks for complications and decline. Many residents have impaired cognition which predisposes them to safety risks and interferes with their ability to communicate symptoms that could aid in detecting complications early.

Family reactions: The guilt, anger, and frustration that families often feel from needing to institutionalize a loved one and watching their loved one decline can be displaced to staff. Expectations may be unrealistic and the realities of the resident's condition may be unaccepted. To complicate matters, family members may have heard horror stories about the awful or abusive conditions in nursing homes and expect that worse.

Staff: Most direct care is provided by nonprofessional caregivers who have minimal education and heavy caseloads. Licensed nurses often are stretched to their limits with multiple clinical and managerial responsibilities. Significant language and cultural differences may exist between residents and staff that can create tension.

Pressures to keep beds filled: Operating a LTCF is an expensive proposition. In order to pay expenses and realize a profit, occupancy needs to be as high as possible. Sometimes, financial pressures will influence admission decisions and residents will be admitted that have more needs than staff realistically can meet with the existing caseload of residents. Likewise, residents who may be problematic may not be discharged or transferred to another facility because of the desire to avoid having empty beds.

A suing society: In a society where people sue because a ladder manufacturer didn't warn them that they'd fall if they placed the ladder in mud or a fast food restaurant didn't advise them that they'd become obese from a steady diet of their burgers, it should come to no surprise that people will be quick to sue a health care facility for a real or suspected wrongdoing.

Knowing that the risk for litigation is high, you need to protect yourself, your staff, and your facility by minimizing those risks. Let's examine some of the specific issues that could present challenges.

Minimizing Legal Risks

Abuse

Abuse is doing or threatening to do physical, psychological, financial, or sexual harm to an individual.

Long-term care facilities are high risk environments for resident abuse. The resident population is a highly dependent one that requires considerable assistance. Many residents are confused and have inappropriate and bothersome behaviors. The frustration and anger residents feel frequently are displaced to staff, who often may be criticized and seldom thanked for their efforts. Staffing problems may cause staff to be overworked and highly stressed. Some staff may have limited education and experience in working with an institutionalized population and may react inappropriately to residents' behaviors and the stress of caregiving. In addition, there may be staff who, in their personal lives, use violence as a way of dealing with conflict.

Although most people think of abuse in terms of beating or grossly neglecting residents, the following also are examples of situations that could constitute abuse:

- A nurse demands money from a resident in return for performing routine care procedures
- A nursing assistant takes a resident's coat, claiming that the resident doesn't have any use for it anyway
- A resident is told that if she soils her clothing again she will be placed in the hallway nude
- A resident is locked in the linen closet to prevent him from wandering away
- A resident who is extremely afraid of snakes is told that there are snakes under her bed
- A resident with dementia regularly curses and strikes at his roommate
- A group of nursing assistants who are bathing a confused resident look on and laugh as one of the assistants plays with the resident's genitalia

Staff should report all cases of real or suspected abuse. Even if a resident's or family member's charge of abuse seems unfounded, it still should be reported and investigated. States may vary in their reporting mechanisms (for example, in some states the licensing division of the health department and the local police are to be notified). Many states have statutes that make it a crime *not* to report resident abuse. Your director of nursing and/or administrator will know the process that needs to be followed, so be sure to report the abuse to them.

The nursing department should have policies and procedures that describe how cases of abuse are investigated, reported, and resolved, and you should be familiar with them. Residents who display problem behaviors should be assessed for their potential to abuse others and strategies planned to prevent their abusive behaviors.

Advance Directives

> *An advance directive is a document expressing a competent individual's choice about care at a future time.*

Advance directives—or, living wills as they are commonly called—give individuals an opportunity to express their opinions about life sustaining measures and have those opinions honored should they become incompetent.

Regulations require that:

> *The resident has a right to a written description of the facility's policies to implement advance directive and applicable State law. If an adult individual is incapacitated at the time of admission and is unable to receive information (due to the incapacitating condition or a mental disorder) or articulate whether or not he or she has executed an advance directive, the facility may give advance directive information to the individual's family or surrogate in the same manner that it issues other materials about policies and procedures to the family of the*

114

incapacitated individual or to a surrogate or other concerned persons in accordance with State law. The facility is not relieved of its obligation to provide this information to the individual once he or she is no longer incapacitated or unable to receive such information.

Virtually all states recognize advance directives. Some states specify formal measures with which the advance directive must comply in order to be binding, and some stipulate the type of form on which this advance directive must be written. To assure that advance directives are recognized as valid, the individuals writing them should adhere to the requirements of their specific states or seek legal counsel. Refer to your facility's policy and procedure regarding advance directives. The advance directive should be placed in the resident's record and all staff involved in the resident's care should be made aware that it exists.

Any opinions expressed by a resident concerning preferences about life sustaining measures should be documented in the resident's record. This information can be of value at a later date in clarifying the resident's desires or offering direction in the absence of an advance directive.

Assault and Battery

Assault *is an intentional threat to cause physical harm by touching a person without his or her consent, whereby the person believes that the threat could be carried out.*

Battery *is the actual act of touching the individual without consent.*

Every individual has the right to privacy and freedom from being touched against his or her will. Assault and battery laws offer people protection in this area.

In the long-term care facility, situations that could cause liability for assault and/or battery include:

- A nursing assistant tells a resident that if he keeps trying to trip staff with his cane, the nursing assistant will take away his cane and hit him over the head with it
- A physician does a skin graft to a resident's pressure ulcer without obtaining the resident's consent to do so
- A resident refuses to have a bath and is forced into the tub by several nursing staff to be given the bath
- A nurse places a strip of adhesive tape over the mouth of a resident who has been screaming curse words at staff
- One nursing assistant forces food into a resident's mouth as another nursing assistant holds the resident's head
- The charge nurse is concerned because an employee has come on duty in what appears to be an intoxicated state and asks the employee to leave the unit. When the employee refuses to leave the nurse grabs the employee by the arm and pulls the employee off the unit.

To reduce the risk of liability for assault and battery charges:

- assure that consent has been obtained for treatments and procedures that are beyond basic care measures
- do not force residents to receive care that they refuse
- allow only employees of the facility or other approved caregivers to provide care for residents
- do not threaten to harm residents or coworkers, even in jest
- never use physical force to remove a coworker or visitor from the facility (call a security officer or the local police)

Competency

More and more long-term care facilities are caring for residents who have altered mental function. When a resident's mental competency is in question, obtaining consent for treatment becomes somewhat more complicated. Legally, when residents are declared by the court to be mentally incompetent, they are not able to legally grant consent. However, the problem for many long-term care facilities is that many of their residents who have questionable mental competency have not been formally declared incompetent by a judicial proceeding.

Assess the mental status of residents upon admission to the facility and periodically thereafter. When changes in mental status are discovered, a comprehensive psychiatric evaluation is helpful in determining competency. If the resident is believed to be mentally incompetent, discuss this with your unit nurse so that action can be taken to have competency determined and a guardian appointed. In most cases, the next of kin is appointed guardian, but since this isn't always the case, the name of the guardian should be clearly indicated in the resident's record.

Confidentiality

Staff have access to an enormous amount of information about residents. Not only data about health status, but information related to finances, family relationships, social problems, and other personal aspects of residents' lives are made available to staff. This information is valuable in gaining an understanding of residents and providing individualized care. However, if staff is careless in the use of this information, legal problems can develop.

Residents have a right to privacy, which includes not having their care and personal information discussed or made known to unauthorized persons. Staff must be careful to respect the confidentiality of information pertaining to residents. Some guidelines that can help staff avoid invasions to residents' privacy include the following:

- Discuss information pertaining to residents only with other staff.
- If asked for personal information about a resident by persons not involved with the resident's care, inform them that you cannot discuss the resident.
- Avoid leaving residents' records, care plans, or notations about residents where they may be seen by visitors or residents.
- Do not give information about residents to telephone callers or via email communication.
- Refer forms requesting information about residents to the appropriate person in the facility; do not complete such forms without authorization.
- Do not discuss residents or events that took place in the facility in public places or within earshot of persons who are not staff.

Consent

Upon admission to a long-term care facility, residents typically sign a consent form that authorizes the facility to perform basic routine and customary services, such as bathing, feeding, and administering medications. When procedures that exceed basic care are required, additional consent must be obtained for each separate procedure; this would include:

- surgery
- diagnostic procedures in which there is more than a slight risk of complications (e.g., myelogram)
- administration of experimental or nonapproved drugs
- radiation therapy
- use of anesthesia

- participation in research
- invasive medical procedures

In general, it is safe for consent to be obtained for any procedure that involves a special explanation to residents or entails more than a minor risk of complications or side effects. When in doubt, it is wise to get consent!

Consent must be informed. **Informed consent** means that the details of the procedure have been thoroughly explained to the resident in a language that the resident can understand. To offer informed consent there should be a description given to the resident of:

- a detailed explanation of the procedure to be performed
- the risks associated with the procedure
- expected outcome
- possible complications that can develop
- alternatives to the procedure

The specific information given to the resident should be documented on the consent form.

The resident should be competent to understand the explanations given and grant or refuse consent. If the resident is believed to be incompetent to grant consent, a judicial procedure to evaluate the resident and appoint a legal guardian should be sought. In some emergency situations, health care professionals can proceed with treatment without the resident's consent or with the consent of the next of kin.

If at any time after granting consent the resident has questions about the procedure, seems to be misinformed about the procedure, or has a change of mind about consenting to the procedure, report this promptly to the unit nurse or physician who plans to do the procedure. It is a sound idea to document this information in the resident's record, also.

Defamation

Communicating—verbally or in writing—a message that injures a person's reputation is considered defamation.
***Libel** refers to the written form of defamation;*
***slander** refers to the oral form.*

Defamation involves making or writing a statement that is harmful to another individual. Saying an injurious statement directly to the individual is not considered defamation; the statement must be made to a third party.

All staff must be careful of statements made about residents and coworkers to avoid charges of defamation. Situations such as the following could make staff liable for defamation:

- The charge nurse, while touring a group of volunteers through the unit, points to a resident and says "You see that resident over there? She was known as quite a wild one in her day. It would not surprise me if she lost her mind due to some venereal disease."
- A nursing assistant tells a visitor that she thinks the son of one of the residents is stealing the resident's money.
- A nurse tells other staff during a conference that she heard the new medical director has a reputation for sexually abusing residents.
- A supervisor tells the director of nursing that she once worked with the nursing assistant that the director just hired and, although it was never proven, she knows that the assistant was a narcotics user.

It is important for all staff to avoid statements that are untrue or based on assumptions rather than facts.

Documentation

The primary purpose of the resident's record is to communicate information about the resident and the resident's care. This information can support claims for reimbursement and offer proof of care provided for future reference. And, you're most likely familiar with the statement: *if it isn't documented, there is no proof it was done.* When staff omit documentation, they not only jeopardize residents' care by neglecting to communicate information about residents' status and services provided, but they also fail to credit themselves for the care they've given.

Staff should be careful not to place unnecessary documentation demands on themselves. For instance, there is no reason for an intake and output record to be maintained on residents who have no problems in this area. Special flowsheets and checklists should be used only when necessary because *once they are initiated, these forms must be maintained accurately by staff.*

Staff needs to understand that the resident's record is a legal document that possibly could be examined in a court of law. Contents of the record, therefore, should be legible, objective, and appropriate.

Do-Not-Resuscitate (DNR) Orders

Legally, a decision not to resuscitate is a decision about medical care, and like other decisions about medical care, requires a physician's order. The fact that the interdisciplinary team discussed the issue at a team conference and agreed that the resident should be categorized DNR does not substitute for the need for an order to exist. *The decision not to resuscitate is a medical decisions that requires a physician's order.*

It is beneficial to discuss the issue of resuscitation with the resident and family at the time of the resident's admission to the facility. If the resident is mentally competent, he or she must consent to the DNR order; if it is believed that this discus-

121

Suggested Guidelines for
Managing Incidents and Accidents:

- Document all unusual occurrences on incident/ accident forms.
- Use the facility's designated form for documenting incidents and accidents as described in the facility's policy manual.
- Complete the incident/accident form as soon as possible after the situation occurred.
- Write legibly and complete all parts of the form.
- Include only observed facts, not opinions. For example, if a resident was found on the floor next to the bed state "Resident found on floor at side of bed" rather than "Resident fell out of bed." If witnesses offer   information related to the event include their comments in quotes rather than having the statements appear as observed facts.
- Do not draw conclusions or make diagnostic statements. For example, rather than stating "Employee pulled back muscle while lifting resident" write instead, "Employee holding back and complaining of lower back pain that he claims began while lifting resident."
- Thoroughly assess the incident/accident victim for injury, even if that person claims to be uninjured.
- Contact your supervisor as soon as possible.
- Seek appropriate help for injured persons and document these efforts on the incident/accident form. If help is refused, document this. For example, "Visitor refused to be transported to hospital and demanded to walk from unit unassisted."
- When even the slightest suspicion of a resident injury exists, have the resident evaluated by a physician or a hospital.
- Forward the incident/accident form to the appropriate office or individual, as designated in the policy.
- Document facts pertaining to the resident's status and actions taken on the resident's record.
- Correct factors that have contributed to incidents and accidents whenever possible.

sion will be detrimental to the resident's well-being, or if the resident is incompetent, consent should be obtained from the legal guardian or family. Documentation of this discussion should exist, indicating that the resident has been informed of and understands his or her prognosis, care and treatment goals, and the resident's desires concerning resuscitation and life sustaining measures.

You should be aware of those residents for whom a DNR order exists and adhere to the facility's policy concerning this order.

False Imprisonment

*Detaining individuals against their will
is considered false imprisonment.*

A mentally competent resident who chooses to leave the facility should not be prevented from doing so. Staff should not lock residents in their rooms or use restraints to limit their movement about the facility or prevent them from leaving the facility. When a resident decides to leave the facility against medical advice, document this information in the resident's record; it may be wise to notify the resident's next of kin or responsible party so that they may intervene and assist the resident. Special provisions do exist for health care facilities to detain residents with communicable diseases or who have mental illnesses that cause them to be a threat to themselves or others. Be sure to contact your supervisor when faced with this type of situation.

Employees should not be detained in the facility against their will, either. Examples in which this could arise could include:

- an employee is suspected of having stolen medications from the drug cart and is attempting to leave the facility. The employee's supervisor has called the local police but

123

wants to keep the employee on the premises so that the drugs can be found on the employee.

- an employee reports to work in what seems to be an intoxicated state with slurred speech and unsteady gait. When questioned about her condition she yells at the charge nurse and says she is leaving. The charge nurse and other staff are concerned that the employee is not able to drive safely and ask her to either stay or wait until they can arrange for her to be driven home. The employee refuses and says she is going to drive herself; coworkers take her car keys from her and prevent her from leaving the break room until a taxi arrives.

Although there appear to be legitimate reason for wanting to detain the employees in the facility, legally, these employees cannot be forced to stay against their will. In situations such as these it is useful to involve security personnel or local police and document the situation completely (describing what was observed, instructions or advice given to the employee, the employee's comments and reactions, witnesses).

Incidents and Accidents

The complex needs of residents, the diversity of personnel, and the many unpredictables that emerge cause incidents and accidents to be realities in the long-term care setting. An **incident** is anything that happens out of the ordinary, such as the loss of personal property, improper administration of a medication, resident or employee slip on the floor, and resident wandering from the facility. An **accident** implies that an unintentional injury has resulted; for example, the resident who was given an improper medication develops a reaction, the person who slipped on the floor has a break in the skin, and the resident who wandered off the premises becomes hypothermic.

All incidents and accidents must be documented on the form

designated by the facility. No matter how minor or insignificant incidents and accidents seem, they need to be documented. The accuracy of the incident and accident documentation can prove invaluable to the facility in the event of litigation.

You should consult with the facility's policy manual as to the recommended method for documenting and filing incident and accident reports. Usually, these reports are not included in the resident's record and are restricted to a limited audience (for example, the administrator, director of nursing, quality assurance coordinator, and insurance carrier). Rather than a statement that an incident occurred, only facts that relate to the resident's care and status should be documented in the resident's record.

Invasion of Privacy

Residents have a right to be free from public view and from having their personal information shared with others. Examples of invasions of a resident's privacy include:
- informing the media of a resident's diagnosis
- using a photograph of a resident in an advertisement for the facility without the resident's consent
- discussing the resident's history with the visitors of another resident
- publishing an article about a resident with the unauthorized use of his name and photograph
- allowing an unauthorized person to read the resident's record or observe the resident's care

Federal regulations do describe requirements in regard to residents' privacy, specifically that residents have the right to:
- approve or release personal and clinical records to outside agencies
- send and receive mail unopened

- receive visitors
- use a telephone in private

Staff should respect and make every effort to assure residents' right to privacy.

Malpractice

When residents enter a long-term care facility they contract for services to be provided, and they rightly expect that these services will meet certain standards. When the standards are not met and harm results to residents as a consequence, malpractice may be charged. Situations that could lead to malpractice include:

- While administering medications, the nurse gives Mr. James Smith's digoxin to Mr. John Smith
- The nursing assistant does not measure the temperature of the water in an enema and uses an excessively hot solution
- A nurse leaves irrigating solution at the bedside of a confused resident, who proceeds to drink it
- An immobile resident does not have her position changed for an entire shift
- Staff notice that a resident is having difficulty breathing and has poor coloring, but forget to notify the physician
- Staff fail to check for several hours the location of a resident who is known to wander
- A nursing assistant who has not been trained to do nasogastric feedings is given this responsibility
- The nurse does not detect an adverse drug reaction

The fact that a resident developed a complication or that staff performed procedures incorrectly does not necessarily mean that malpractice exists, thus the above examples may not result in liability. For staff to be liable for malpractice these conditions must be present:

Duty: A relationship exists between residents and staff

whereby residents are contracting for services to be provided and staff is being paid to perform those services.

Negligence: An action fails to be meet the acceptable standard for that action.

Injury: Harm results as a result of the negligent action.

Malpractice may not exist if a staff member took an inappropriate action but no harm resulted, for example, if Mr. John Smith was administered Mr. James Smith's digoxin but had no ill effect. Likewise, if a resident developed a complication but it was not related to a staff action, it may be difficult to prove malpractice.

Tips for Reducing Malpractice Risks

- Be familiar with and follow the accepted policies and procedures of the facility
- Consult with the physician when there is an order that is unclear or seems inappropriate
- Know residents' normal status and promptly report changes in their status
- Follow-up on the status of laboratory tests; promptly report the results of laboratory and other diagnostic tests to the physician
- Do not accept responsibilities that are beyond your capabilities to perform and do not delegate assignments unless you know staff is competent to do them
- Read residents' care plans and orders before giving care
- Discuss with supervisors assignments that cannot be completed due to insufficient staff or supplies
- Report broken equipment and other safety hazards
- Check residents' armbands and validate their identities before giving care to them

- Report and/or file an incident report when unusual situations occur
- Document observations about residents' status, care given, and other information about residents and care activities
- Attend educational programs and keep current of knowledge and skills pertaining to your job

Restraints

The Omnibus Budget Reconciliation Act (OBRA) placed new emphasis on the cautious use of restraints in its statement that:

the resident has the right to be free from physical or
chemical restraints imposed for the purposes of discipline
or convenience and not required to treat
the resident's medical condition

Restraints are to be used only for the physical safety of the resident or other residents, and must be accompanied by a physician's order that specifies the duration and circumstances under which the restraints are to be used.

Anything that restricts the resident's movement is considered a restraint and can include:

protective vests
geri-chairs
trays on wheelchairs
safety bars
bedrails
safety belts
medications used to control behavior

Restraints should be used only after other non-restraining alternatives have proven unsuccessful. There should be detailed documentation describing the other approaches used.

Improperly used restraints can lead to litigation for false imprisonment and negligence associated with resident injury and death. To avoid such consequences, nursing staff should pay attention to the following guidelines:

Prior to using restraints:

- Describe the specific behaviors that the resident demonstrates that pose a risk to the resident or other residents
- Assess the reasons for the behaviors and arrange treatment to improve the resident's behaviors if possible
- Try measures other than restraints to manage the resident's behavior; such measures could include alarm systems on doors, wristband alarms, bed alarm pads, bean bag pillows, and beds and chairs that are close to floor level
- Evaluate the effectiveness of alternative measures
- Describe the amount of risk the resident poses to himself and others by not being restrained

When restraints are deemed necessary:

- Contact your supervisor to discuss obtaining a physician's order for the restraint; this order should describe the conditions for which the restraint should be used, type of restraint, and duration of use
- Maintain a flowsheet or other charting system that describes when the restraint was begun, times released/changed, resident's response, and effectiveness
- Closely observe the restrained resident
- Adhere to the facility's policies and procedures for the use of restraints
- Regularly re-evaluate the need for the restraint
- Document all of the above in the resident's record

It must be reinforced that the use of restraints carry considerable risks to residents and the facility. In addition to restraints potentially causing injury and even death to residents, restraints significantly compromise the freedom of residents and further limit their function. Restraints should be considered a last resort, after all other alternative measures have been judged to be ineffective.

Supervisory Responsibility

In the long-term care facility, supervisors/managers often assume significant responsibility. Many different employees may be under a team leader's responsibility. Liability can result for negligence in carrying out supervisory responsibilities in situations such as:

- assigning tasks to employees that are not within the employees' job descriptions or scope of practice
- delegating tasks to employees when you are aware that the employees have not been trained to do the tasks
- failing to correct the incompetent performance of subordinates
- allowing employees to work who you know are incompetent or dangerous

You need to be familiar with the competencies and qualifications of the staff for whom you are responsible. Even if subordinates are believed to be qualified and competent, observation and evaluation of subordinates' performance during the shift are essential. Be sure to make your supervisor aware of employees who you believe are incompetent or dangerous and who have not responded to corrective actions.

Telephone Orders

Most long-term care facilities do not have physicians on site 24 hours each day, therefore, nursing staff must rely on telephone communication to inform physicians of changes in the status of residents and to receive instructions from physicians.

In the event that a physician does not respond to a telephone call within a reasonable time, seek other actions to assist the resident. For example, consult with your supervisor about contacting the medical director, another physician, or the administrator. If you assess the resident's condition to be in jeopardy or in need of prompt attention you have a responsibility to arrange transfer of the resident to a local hospital. Documenting "message left with physician's office concerning resident's status" or "physician notified" does not relieve nurses of intervening and seeking treatment for residents who present a medical emergency.

Some recommendations that can aid in reducing the risks associated with telephone orders are offered on the next page.

Guidelines for Telephone Orders

• Follow your facility's policy and procedure regarding who may telephone physicians and accept telephone orders.

• Assess the resident prior to the telephone communication and have the assessment data readily available during the conversation.

• Inform the physician of the resident's current status, vital signs, and significant observations. Remind the physician of the medications currently being administered to the resident.

• If you are given the responsibility of communicating with they physician, speak directly to the physician, not through an office nurse or other staff.

• Write the order as it is being given and read it back to the physician (if your facility allows you to accept telephone orders).

• If possible, have the physician fax the order to you.

• Question orders that seem unsafe or inappropriate. If the physician demands that the order be followed despite your objection, inform the physician that you will not implement the order until you can verify it with your supervisor.

• Write the entire order on the order sheet, identifying it as a telephone order. Sign your name.

• Remind the physician to sign the order within 24 hours.

Chapter 7

GROWING IN YOUR ROLE

It wouldn't be surprising if after reading through this book you begin to think that being a LPN in a long-term care facility is very complex business. And, you're not off target with this view. Although some people think that it is a piece of cake to work in a LTCF, the reality is that it requires that nurses:
- have many clinical and management skills
- know the unique regulations that apply to LTCFs
- be able to function in highly independent roles without having many professionals nearby
- be comfortable with long-term relationships with residents and their families
- have the ability to help care for residents' total needs: physical, emotional, social, and spiritual.

These realities can make LTC nursing an exciting specialty that allows you to use a wide range of knowledge and skills, and to grow in your role. However, these demands also can be highly stressful, so it is important that you actively learn to take care of yourself.

Stress Management
Sources of Stress

LTCFs are particularly stressful places to work due to:

133

- Inability to reverse or improve the conditions of most residents
- Behavioral problems of residents
- Physical care demands of residents
- Repetitious nature of work
- Limited number of staff
- Expectations of residents' families
- Displaced feelings of residents and their families
- Negative image of nursing homes held by public
- Regulatory requirements
- Close monitoring by regulatory agencies (inspections!)
- Frequency of deaths
- Ethical dilemmas

These sources of stress are *chronic* ones, from which LTCF staff is seldom relieved. Chronic stress can have more serious effects than occasional stress. In this light, long-term care nursing is equally stressful to critical care and other nursing specialties.

Effects of Stress

When first confronted with stress, the body mobilizes its defenses and prepares for "fight or flight" with the process show in Display 7-1.

Chronic stress causes the body and mind to be in a state of high alert for an extended period of time, and like an overtaxed machine, this extra workload takes its toll. Symptoms include: insomnia, fatigue, accident proneness, irritability, depression, poor concentration, increased use of sarcasm, complaining, forgetfulness, errors, inattention to detail, reduced productivity, low morale, dissatisfaction with work, and relationship problems.

Display 7-1
Effects of Stress

The sympathetic nervous system is aroused and stimulates the
pituitary gland which releases
ACTH (adrenocorticotropic hormone).

$\downarrow$

The amount of adrenalin in the body rises,
causing an increased state of alertness and
heightening of heart, lung, and muscle activities.

$\downarrow$

As more blood is sent to the muscles, the hands,
fingers, and toes become cold. The pupils dilate and
hearing becomes more acute.

$\downarrow$

Glycogen converts to glucose, blood clotting
increases, and immune reactions are suppressed.

The body's reactions to stress allow it to manage the additional demands it faces. As the stress is eliminated or the
body adapts to it, bodily functions return to normal or near
normal levels.

Managing Stress

Stress is costly. It increases the risk for illness and may
cause behaviors that can lead to serious problems, such as resident abuse or poor job performance. For the facility, stress can
increase staff turnover and threaten the quality of services provided. And for residents, stress can result in less personalized
care and a lower quality of life. It is essential that you make

Helpful Measures for Personal Stress Management

- Evaluate and attempt to change sources of stress
- Learn to manage time effectively
- Limit your overtime
- Discuss and try to solve problems with coworkers
- Try not to personalize criticisms from residents and families. Remember the situation is the problem, although you may be the target of displaced emotions
- Rotate assignments of residents who are difficult to care for
- Recognize the symptoms of stress in yourself and seek the help of an objective party to assist you in discussing and managing your feelings
- Learn techniques for controlling your response to stress (e.g., deep breathing, repeating a word, saying a prayer, counting to 25)
- Withdraw from the situation and seek help when you feel you may lose control
- When you feel "burned out" or as though you cannot cope, request time off
- Instead of coffee and cigarette breaks, enjoy breaks in which you do short relaxation exercises, recline in a quiet area, or listen to relaxation tapes
- Eat a well-balanced diet; avoid junk foods
- Regularly exercise
- Do something for yourself to unwind between work and home
- Take naps; allow ample time for sleep
- Schedule leisure activities into your life; develop a hobby
- Do not rely on cigarettes, alcohol, or drugs to assist in relaxation
- Learn about meditation and relaxation exercises, and build them into your life

stress management an essential part of your self-care practices. Some measures that could prove helpful are offered on the next page.

You and many of your staff leave a day's work of caring for residents to go home and begin the work of caring for families. This offers little opportunity for job-related stress to be eliminated before home/family-related stress begins. A special effort must be made to unwind and relieve stress before assuming home responsibilities. Measures that can assist this effort include:

- taking a short walk in a mall or park
- sitting in a warm bathtub of water
- napping
- sitting in a quiet room in which there is aromatherapy with the scent of lavender and listening to relaxing music
- performing meditation or relaxation exercises
- reading a magazine or book

Just 15 minutes of uninterrupted personal private time can aid in recharging yours batteries and providing the physical and emotional energy needed to face home responsibilities.

Minor changes in the work environment can aid in reducing stress. For example, aromatherapy using the scent of lavender can be relaxing and pleasant. Noise control and playing relaxing music can be beneficial (special soundtracks for stress-reduction and nature sounds are available). Encouraging staff to do stretching exercises and deep breathing, or partnering with a coworker for a seated, clothed back massage can promote relaxation. As a special benefit, some facilities contract with massage therapists to provide massages to staff during their work day.

Every individual needs to develop a lifestyle that strengthens the ability to manage stress. This begins with good, basic health practices such as eating a sensible diet, exercising, and getting adequate rest. Leisure activities are a necessary component of a healthy lifestyle; time should be scheduled in busy lives for hobbies, sports, and other recreational activities. Of course, risk factors such as cigarette smoking, high caffeine consumption, inappropriate use of drugs, and lack of regular exercise weaken the ability to manage stress.

Continuing Education

New drugs and technology...different ways to treat illnesses...added responsibilities...increased litigation.... Health and medical care have changed through the years–in some cases, very dramatically–and will continue to do so. No nurse, physician, or other health care professional can expect to practice throughout his or her career without learning new knowledge and skills. Continuing education is essential if you want to stay competent.

Some of your continuing education needs can be met through your facility's staff development program. Typically, inservice education programs will review topics that are common to the LTCF (e.g., infection control, resident rights, fire safety) and teach you about new procedures and policies.

As you assume new or expanded responsibilities, you may need additional training. This may be able to be obtained within your facility through individualized training sessions or mentoring. Sometimes, you may need to attend programs outside your facility.

It is a good idea to try to attend workshops outside your facility periodically. This helps you to gain new perspectives from those of your employing facility and helps you to meet other nurses with whom you can network. Large conferences are great places to not only attend workshops, but to see new products that are exhibited. Nursing associations and publica-

138

tions for nurses are good sources to learn about these opportunities

Busy schedules and scarce funds can limit the workshops you may be able to attend, but you still can commit to your education through self-study. Independent study courses, internet programs, and continuing education articles in nursing journals are good sources of affordable self-study programs.

In addition to continuing education, you should consider education for career advancement. Advancing to a registered nurse is a logical step for you, and one that you are very prepared for. The additional education will pave the way for you to have more career opportunities and more earnings. You can contact local community colleges or universities to learn about their nursing   programs. Even if you start taking one course a year, you will be on your path of getting that degree!

Your Special Contribution

As has been pointed out many times, working in a LTCF is not easy work. It usually doesn't bring a great deal of recognition, compliments, or earnings. And, it is physically and emotionally demanding. With all that said, LTC nursing *is* a very important specialty. To provide competent, compassionate care to those who are too disabled or old to care for themselves–particularly in a society that tends to undervalue these individuals–is sacred work. On behalf of those who have benefited from your nursing and those who may in the future, thank you for all you do. May your work and life be blessed for your special commitment and contribution.

INDEX